T0359478

POCKET GUIDE TO

ECGs

Duncan Guy
BMedSci, MB BS, PhD, FRACP

The McGraw·Hill Companies

Sydney New York San Francisco Auckland
Bangkok Bogotá Caracas Hong Kong
Kuala Lumpur Lisbon London Madrid
Mexico City Milan New Delhi San Juan
Seoul Singapore Taipei Toronto

First edition published 2002
Second edition published 2006
Second revised edition published 2012

Copyright © 2012 McGraw-Hill Australia Pty Limited
Additional owners of copyright are acknowledged in on-page credits.

Every effort has been made to trace and acknowledge copyrighted material. The authors and publishers tender their apologies should any infringement have occurred.

National Library of Australia Cataloguing-in-Publication Data

Author:	Guy, Duncan.
Title:	Pocket guide to ECGs / Duncan Guy.
Edition:	2nd ed. revised
ISBN:	9781743070680 (pbk.)
Subjects:	Electrocardiography. Electrodiagnosis.
Dewey Number:	616.1207547

Published in Australia by
McGraw-Hill Australia Pty Ltd
Level 2, 82 Waterloo Road, North Ryde NSW 2113
Publisher: Fiona Richardson
Production editor: Natalie Crouch
Proofreader: Vicki Deakin
Indexer: Mary Coe
Cover design: Patricia McCallum and Dominic Giustarini
Internal design: Patricia McCallum
Typeset in 8.5 pt Palatino_Light by diacriTech
Printed in China on 95 gsm matt art by 1010 Printing International Limited

CONTENTS

INTRODUCTION

The ECG is one of the most common tests we perform to assist us to reach an accurate clinical assessment of our patients. It is a piece of the overall clinical jigsaw puzzle but, like a piece in a puzzle, the ECG on its own rarely gives us the full picture. Three overall principles will ensure an accurate conclusion is made from an ECG:

1. Include the history and examination findings in your deliberation when looking at an ECG.
2. Do not jump to the first and most obvious diagnosis; always follow a systematic method for reviewing an ECG.
3. If the interpretation of a finding on the ECG is not clear, return to the patient and take a more thorough history. Extra information often clarifies the place of the ECG in the overall clinical puzzle.

Without an adequate clinical history, physical examination and other investigations, an ECG rarely gives us the full clinical picture and it is with this caveat that isolated ECGs should be interpreted. The aim of this book is to provide you with the skills and methods to glean as much information as possible from an ECG so that it can be accurately placed in the clinical puzzle.

THIS BOOK

The ECG is a recording of the electrical activity of the heart. It is one of the most widely performed cardiac investigations. The skill of accurately interpreting an ECG is one that is easily acquired when armed with the correct information, a thorough interpretation sequence and the time and persistence to practise the skills. This handbook will provide you with the information and a method of accurate interpretation; the practice is up to you!

The handbook is divided into four sections. The first section gives you details about the normal ECG, including how to record an ECG and details on the normal intervals. It also outlines a stepwise method for interpreting an ECG. The second section details common abnormalities encountered in each of the interpretation steps detailed in Section 1. This allows you to use Section 1 to assist with reviewing an ECG; if part of the ECG is abnormal you can use the index link at the bottom of the page to refer to the appropriate part of Section 2 to diagnose common abnormalities.

Section 3 contains an overview of common ECG abnormalities that can be used as a reference.

Section 4 contains an overview of the interpretation of ECGs in patients with a pacemaker and the ECG changes pacemakers can produce.

The paragraphs introduced by ✐ (e.g. see 'Sinus tachycardia' on p. 37) contain new information and tips relevant to the topic and to real daily practice.

The access to the website included with the book is an interactive self-learning tool for students and practitioners. It presents basic and advanced ECGs via interactive cases, which explain each step of the interpretation. The cases combine the clinical history with an ECG and the interactive step-by-step learning method. At the end of each case there are questions to consider and links to the theory to assist in learning about ECGs in a clinical context. This pragmatic, interactive and clinically-based learning method makes this online resource extremely relevant to every-day practice. In addition, the website is constantly being improved. Any updates are immediately available to any registered users of this resource.

ABOUT THE AUTHOR

Dr Duncan Guy, BMedSci, MB BS, PhD, FRACP, is a cardiologist practising at Castle Hill and Westmead in Sydney, Australia. He is also CEO of Specialist Services Medical Group. www.specialistservices.com.au

ACKNOWLEDGMENTS

The science and art of interpretation of the ECG are learnt and refined over many years of training. I am indebted to the many physicians and colleagues who have taught me this skill, in particular, the cardiologists of Westmead Hospital.

THE NORMAL ECG

GENERAL ADVICE ON INTERPRETING ECGs

An ECG no different to other tests done in medicine. It is only really accurate and useful when placed into a clinical context. The most important part of interpreting an ECG is taking a history and examining the patient before recording the ECG. The ECG should not be thought of as a crystal ball that will reveal all–it is a helpful tool that assists with solving clinical puzzles–not the answer.

Many ECG machines now offer computer generated reports. These can be helpful, but remember they are algorithms designed give you a list of possible diagnoses and hence can over-report. Keep in mind that the computer hasn't taken a history or examined the patient–so its chance of being clinically accurate is a less than yours!

Finally if the ECG you are looking at just doesn't seem to make sense–ask a colleague–or fax or email it to a Cardiologist for an opinion. If those options aren't available go with your clinical judgment and do what is the safest option for the patient—even if this means sending them to a hospital for what may be 'nothing'. In all our careers we send a few patients to hospital for 'nothing' to make sure you pick up the 'somethings'.

ECG STANDARD CONVENTIONS

Internationally, ECGs are recorded using the same calibration techniques and background grid. The first step in reviewing any ECG is to confirm that these conventions were adhered to during the recording process. Any variation in the recording method must be taken into account during interpretation.

Calibration signal
A calibration signal should be recorded on all ECGs. For an ECG recorded on the normal settings this signal is 5 mm (l large square, 0.2 s) wide and 10 mm (2 large squares, 1 mV) high.

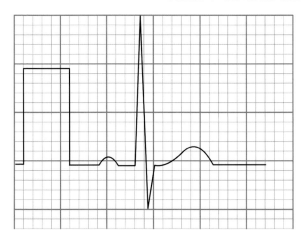

Normal calibration

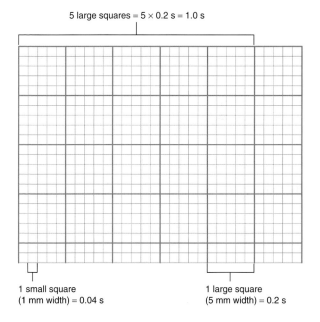

5 large squares = 5 × 0.2 s = 1.0 s

1 small square
(1 mm width) = 0.04 s

1 large square
(5 mm width) = 0.2 s

Paper speed (horizontal calibration)

The ECG grid paper moves through the machine at a standard 25 mm per second. Each small square on the paper is 1 mm, which at this paper speed equals 0.04 seconds (1/25th of a second). Each large square is 5 mm and therefore equals 0.2 seconds. Using this knowledge we can calculate the patient's heart rate and ECG intervals. It is possible to alter the paper speed, usually done by accident, thus altering the interpretation. The width of the calibration signal reflects the paper speed; hence, if the paper is set to double speed (50 mm/s), the signal is double width (2 large squares, 0.4 s). The intervals thus measured on the ECG will all need to be halved to obtain correct values. The opposite applies if the paper speed is halved and the calibration signal is only half a large square wide. The paper in this case is set to 12.5 mm/s and all measured values will need to be doubled to obtain correct readings.

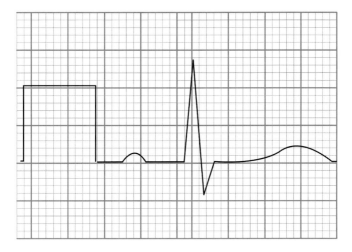

Double paper speed (50 mm/s)

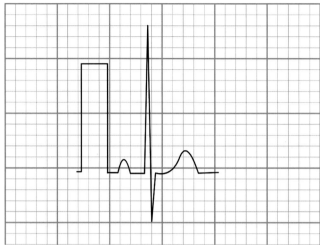

Half paper speed (12.5 mm/s)

Signal height (vertical calibration)

In vertical calibration, 10 mm height represents 1 mV of electrical signal. This gives us a standard calibration signal of 10 mm high. The height of the components of the ECG gives us a guide to the size and wall thickness of the cardiac chambers. Hence, to come to an accurate conclusion, we must be certain the calibration is correct. Some ECG machines will automatically halve the calibration (making it 5 mm to 1 mV) if it records a high QRS signal. If the reviewer of the ECG does not see this reduction in calibration, it may lead to a diagnosis of normal QRS height when in fact there is left ventricular hypertrophy by voltage height criteria.

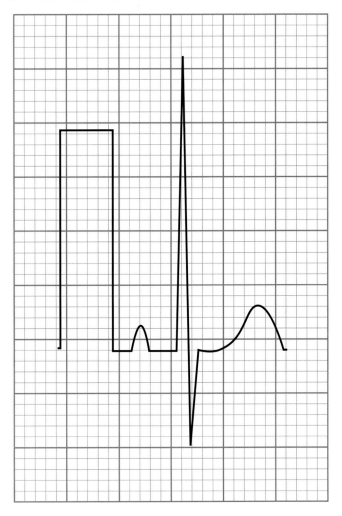

Double signal height

Baseline

The baseline, or isoelectric line, of the ECG is taken as the segment between the end of a T wave and the start of the following P wave. Deflections above this line are regarded as positive and those below are regarded as negative.

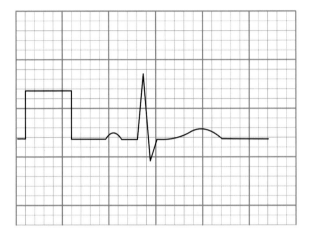

Half signal height

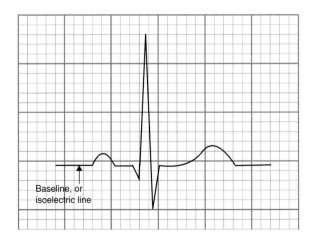

Baseline, or
isoelectric line

Naming conventions for the 'squiggles' of an ECG

- **P wave.** This is a small hump that occurs prior to the larger QRS complex and reflects atrial depolarisation. P waves are not always present and are occasionally not visible in all leads.
- **Q wave.** If the first deflection in the QRS complex is downward it is called a Q wave. Q waves are not always present as seen in the RS complex on page 9. However the conventional terminology used by clinicians and used throughout this book is the QRS complex, even when a Q wave may be absent.
- **R wave.** Any upward deflection in the QRS is called an R wave. It may be preceded by a Q wave or it may be the first deflection of the QRS from the baseline. In some ventricular conduction disorders there can be two R waves in the QRS complex.
- **S wave.** This is a downward deflection occurring *after* the R wave. If there is no R wave, there cannot be an S wave. A downward deflection with no R wave preceding it is, therefore, a Q wave.
- **T wave.** This is a broad hump occurring after the QRS complex and signifies ventricular repolarisation.

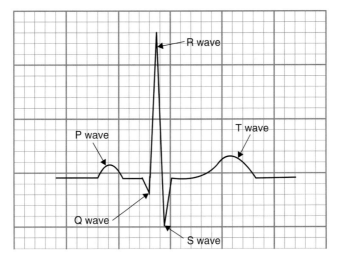

A QRS complex

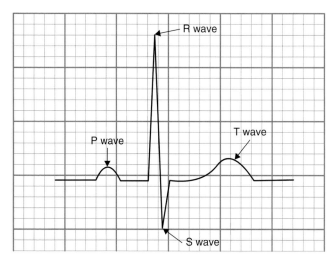

An RS complex

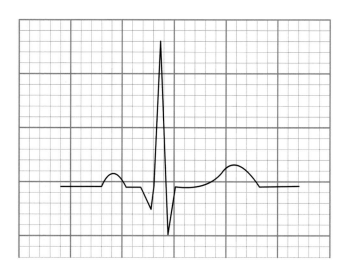

A pathological Q wave

RECORDING LEAD POSITIONS

Standard positions are used for the recording of all ECGs. It is important that the leads are placed in the correct positions as incorrect lead placement will change the ECG signal and may lead to an incorrect diagnosis.

Limb leads

The limb leads are attached to both arms and both legs. In the case of a patient who is an amputee they are placed on the extremity nearest to the normal position.

The right and left arm and left leg leads are active recording leads. The right leg lead is used by the ECG machine as a ground or reference lead. From these three active leads we get six of the recordings of a 12 lead ECG.

- **Lead I** is a recording of the electrical potential difference between right and left arms.
- **Lead II** is a recording of the electrical potential difference between the right arm and left leg.
- **Lead III** is a recording of the electrical potential difference between the left arm and left leg.

Based on recordings from the limb leads, the ECG machine calculates the leads aVF, aVR and aVL. The 'a' stands for *augmented* limb leads.

The limb leads represent the electrical activity of the heart in the vertical plane.

Chest leads

Leads V1 to V6 are the chest leads. They are placed in standard positions across the chest wall and provide us with information on the heart's electrical activity in the horizontal plane (at 90° to the limb leads).

- **V1** is placed on the 4th intercostal space on the right of the sternum (patient's right).
- **V2** is placed on the 4th intercostal space on the left of the sternum.
- **V3** is placed between V2 and V4.
- **V4** is placed on the 5th intercostal space in the mid-clavicular line.
- **V5** is placed at the same level as V4 in the anterior axillary line.
- **V6** is placed at the same level as V4 in the mid-axillary line.

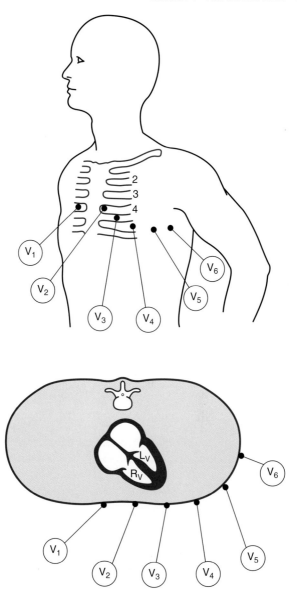

Area of the heart	Leads
Inferior wall	II, III, aVF
Anterior wall	V1 to V4
Lateral wall	V5, V6 and I and aVL
Posterior wall	V1 to V3 can be used to assess the posterior wall

Common recording artifacts

- **Arm lead reversal.** The sign that the arm leads may have been reversed during recording (right arm lead on left arm and vice versa) is that lead aVR is positive. This is accompanied by an abnormal frontal plane axis.
- **Skeletal muscle tremor** is another common artifact in the baseline of the ECG. Patients should be encouraged to relax as much as practical during recording. In the case of patients with an involuntary tremor such as Parkinson's disease, some degree of tremor artifact is expected.
- **Electrical interference** is sometimes recorded by ECG machines as a 50 hertz baseline artifact. Many ECG machines have a filter to remove this, so always ensure it is turned on. If the artifact persists, turn off other electrical devices in the room that may be creating the artifact.

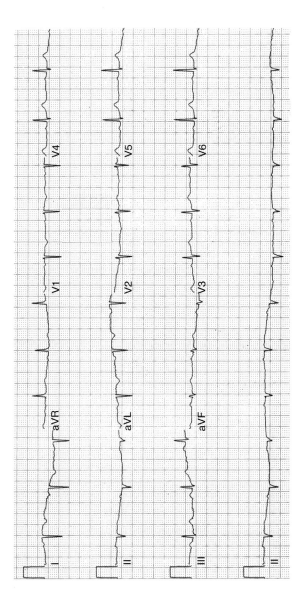

Arm lead reversal

Skeletal muscle tremor

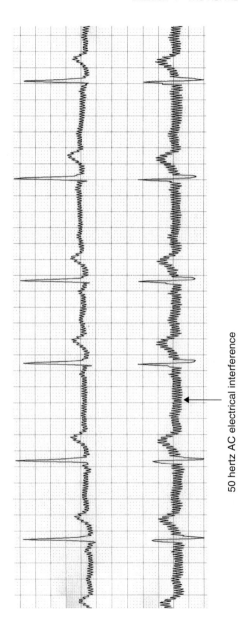

50 hertz AC electrical interference

Electrical interference

STEPS IN INTERPRETATION OF AN ECG AND NORMAL VALUES

Reaching an accurate and thorough conclusion is usually a process of putting together the many pieces of an ECG jigsaw. The following is a sequence that should be used for all ECG interpretation, even when on first glance there is an obvious abnormality. The full and accurate diagnosis is almost never reached by looking at one piece of the ECG puzzle.

1. Regularity in timing of the cardiac rhythm

Looking at the rhythm strip, determine whether the atrial and then ventricular rhythms are:

a. regular
b. regular with occasional irregular beats
c. totally irregular.

Why is it important?

Looking at the regularity of cardiac rhythm allows us to determine whether it comes from one dominant focus or circuit (regular), whether there is a dominant focus but other foci occasionally intervene (regular with occasional irregular beats) or whether the cardiac rhythm originates at multiple sites (totally irregular). Different disorders of rhythm are in each group.

Method

Mark four successive complexes on a piece of paper. Move the paper along the rhythm strip to the next four complexes. If the subsequent complexes fall on the marks you have made on your paper then the rhythm is regular. If there is an occasional beat that doesn't fit the pattern then you have a regular rhythm with occasional irregular beats. A totally irregular pattern will not match your marks. If you are still unsure, mark a larger sample of beats for comparison.

> CLINICAL TIP
>
> It is normal to have some small variation in the heart rate during sinus rhythm with respiration, especially in younger people. This is referred to as *sinus arrhythmia*.

For a discussion of causes of changes in rhythm see Section 2, page 37.

2. Rate

The heart rate is calculated using the underlying grid as the reference. It is important to measure both the atrial rate (if P waves are
evident) and the ventricular rate (using the QRS complexes).

Why is it important?

Heart rate helps us to triage into bradycardia (slow), normal or
tachycardia (fast). Determining the heart rate is also the first step in
diagnosing many rhythm disorders.

Method

There are two methods for calculating the heart rate depending on
whether the rate is regular or irregular.

- **Regular rhythms:** count the number of large squares between
  one QRS complex or P wave and the next. Divide 300 by this number and you will have the rate in beats per minute.
  (Each large square is 0.2 seconds: 300×0.2 seconds $= 60$ seconds.
  Dividing 300 by the number of squares between two complexes
  gives the beats per minute; e.g. three squares between complexes is
  a heart rate of 100 beats per minute.)
- **Irregular rhythms:** when the rhythm is irregular mark 15 large
  squares (remember, each large square is 0.2 seconds duration, thus
  15×0.2 seconds $= 3$ seconds) and then count the number of complexes in that section of the rhythm strip. Multiply the number of
  complexes by 20 to get the heart rate per minute. For example: if
  there were four QRS complexes every 15 large squares, the ventricular rate is approximately 80 per minute (4×20).

CLINICAL TIP

If the heart rate appears profoundly slow, check the calibration
signal and paper speed on which the ECG is recorded. If the paper
is set to a faster speed, the interval between beats and all other
intervals will be abnormally long. Adjust the rates in your report to
compensate for the recording error.

---

*For a discussion of changes in heart rate, see Section 2,
page 36.*

Number of large squares between complexes	Corresponding heart rate
1	300 per minute
2	150 per minute
3	100 per minute
4	75 per minute
5	60 per minute
6	50 per minute

3. P waves

P waves are the ECG representation of atrial depolarisation. They are a combination of right and left atrial depolarisation.

Why is it important?

P waves give us a guide to the size of the atria and whether the atrial rhythm is coming from the sinus node or a non-sinus atrial focus.

What is normal?

Normal values:

a. Duration 0.08 to 0.11 seconds (2 to 3 small squares)
b. Height < 0.25 mV (< 2.5 small squares).

Normal appearance in different leads:

a. Positive in I, II and V2–V6
b. Negative in aVR
c. Biphasic appearance in V1 (*biphasic* means that, relative to the baseline, the P wave has a positive and a negative component)
d. Variable appearance in III.

CLINICAL TIP

If the P waves do not have the normal appearance in different leads, they may be coming from a non-sinus node atrial ectopic pacemaker. The axis of the P waves will help determine from where in the atria they are originating.

For a discussion of abnormal P waves, see Section 2, page 55.

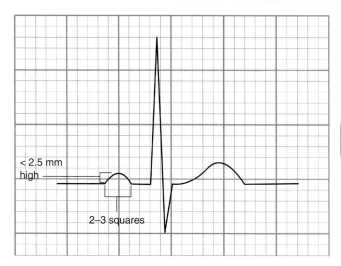

< 2.5 mm high

2–3 squares

The normal P wave

4. Relationship between the P waves and QRS complexes

The relationship between the P waves and QRS complexes gives us information about the sequence of depolarisation in the heart and the site of the dominant pacemaker.

Why is it important?

It is important to determine the site of the dominant pacemaker. This helps us determine the underlying rhythm.

What is normal?

The normal sequence is that all QRS complexes on the ECG are preceded by a P wave. There should only be one P wave per QRS complex and the atrial rate should be the same as the ventricular rate.

CLINICAL TIP

If you cannot see any P waves and the rhythm is regular, be sure to check for them just after the QRS complex or in the T wave. If the rhythm originates in the atrioventricular junction or ventricle, sometimes P waves are found after the QRS.

For a discussion of causes of abnormal P–QRS relationships, see Section 2, page 57.

5. PR interval

The PR interval is measured from the start of the P wave to the start of the QRS or RS complex. It is caused by the delay in conduction from the onset of atrial depolarisation to the onset of ventricular depolarisation.

Why is it important?

The PR interval reflects the time taken for depolarisation to spread from the initial depolarisation of atrial muscle to the start of ventricular muscle depolarisation. The majority of the PR interval is caused by the slow conduction through the atrioventricular node. Disease or short circuit of any of these parts of the conduction system are shown as abnormalities of the PR interval.

What is normal?

Measured from the start of the P wave to the onset of the QRS or RS complex the PR interval should be between 0.12 and 0.20 seconds (3 to 5 small squares).

CLINICAL TIP

The segment from the end of the P wave to the start of the QRS or RS complex is called the PR segment and reflects the time taken for the impulse to cross the atrioventricular junction and enter the His-Purkinje system in the ventricle. This segment should be ≤ 3 small squares (0.12 s).

For a discussion of an abnormal PR interval, see Section 2, page 57.

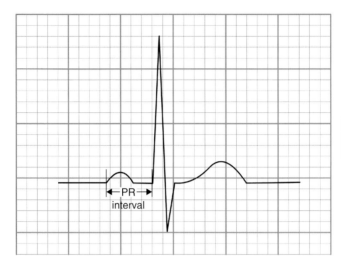

The normal PR interval

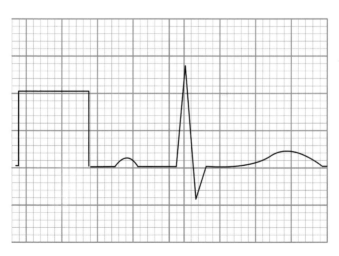

Normal PR interval recorded on double paper speed (50 mm/s)

6. Q wave

The Q wave is an initial negative (downwards) deflection from the baseline after the P wave. Q waves are not always present. It can be either a normal finding or pathological, depending on the clinical circumstances and the recording leads in which it appears.

What is normal?

Q waves can be regarded as normal if they appear in only lead III and/or aVR. In the other leads they can usually be regarded as normal when they are either less than 1 mm wide and 1 mm deep, or less than 25% of the R wave in size.

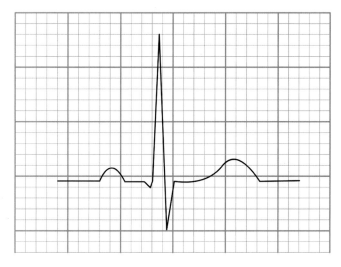

A non-pathological Q wave

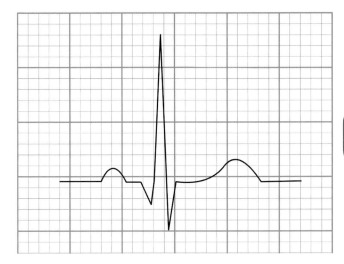

A pathological Q wave

CLINICAL TIP

If a Q wave is seen only in lead III, it is helpful to record this lead again after the patient has taken a deep breath in. Often the Q wave will have disappeared, confirming that it is not a pathological finding.

7. QRS width

The width of the QRS complex is a measurement of the time taken from onset to completion of ventricular depolarisation. The width of the QRS complex reflects the time delay from arrival of the depolarisation wavefront in the ventricle to total depolarisation of both ventricles.

Why is it important?

The width of the QRS reflects the conduction of the electrical wavefront through the bundle of His and its branches via the Purkinje fibres to the ventricular myocardium.

What is normal?

Measured from the first deviation from the baseline after the P wave to the end of the S wave the normal width is < 3 small squares (0.08–0.12 s).

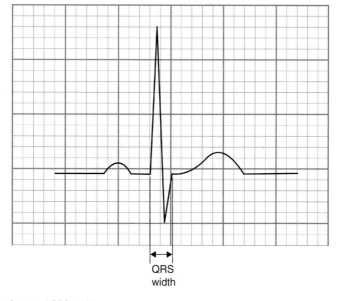

QRS
width

A normal QRS width

For a discussion of abnormal QRS width, see Section 2, page 66.

1

8. R wave

An R wave is any positive (upwards) deflection of the QRS complex. It is caused by the wave of ventricular depolarisation spreading towards the recording electrode.

What is normal?

The R wave should increase in size from V2 across to V4 or V5. It may be absent in lead V1 and/or aVR; this can be normal.

The size of the R wave depends on two factors:

1. **Ventricular muscle mass.** The greater the ventricular wall thickness, the larger the electrical signal generated and hence the greater the deflection on the ECG (R wave).
2. **The distance of the recording electrode from the heart.** If the electrode is very close to the heart, as occurs in very thin people or pectus excavatum, the R waves are large. If the electrodes are distant to the heart, as occurs in pericardial effusion or morbid obesity, the R waves are smaller.

The size of the R wave is usually measured in V5 or V6 and should be < 25 mm in older individuals and < 30 mm in younger thin people.

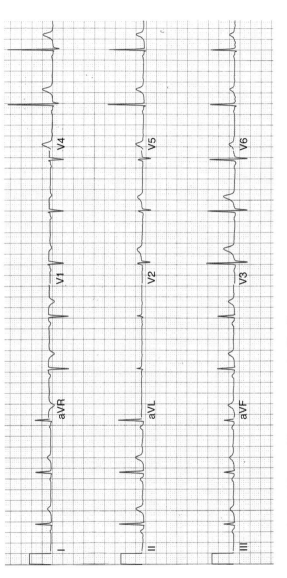

Normal sinus rhythm with normal R wave progression V1→V6

9. S wave

The S wave is a negative deflection in the QRS or RS complex occurring after an R wave. The point at which it ends is termed the J point. It is caused by the wave of ventricular depolarisation spreading away from the recording electrode.

What is normal?

The S wave is usually deepest in V1 and decreases in size across to V5 and V6 where it can be absent. The S wave in V1 or V2 should be < 25 mm deep when measured from the isoelectric line.

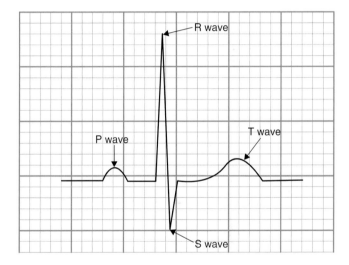

An RS complex

CLINICAL TIP

The summation of the size of the R wave in V6 and the S wave in V2, or the R wave in V5 and the S wave in V1, is used as a criterion for assessing the presence of left ventricular hypertrophy on the ECG.

10. J point
The J point is the point in each QRS-T complex where the QRS changes to an ST segment. The movement of the complex changes from predominantly vertical to horizontal. This turning point is the J point. It is used as a reference point for assessing ST segments.

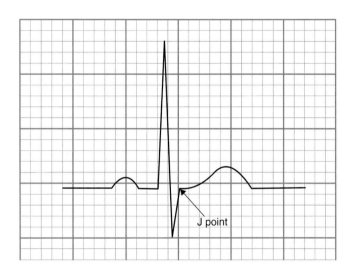

11. ST segment
The ST segment is the interval between the end of the QRS complex (J point) and the onset of the T wave. It is a segment of unchanged net polarisation of ventricular muscle, and signifies the period between the end of depolarisation and the onset of repolarisation.

What is normal?
The ST segment should be level with the baseline (isoelectric). It is regarded as elevated when it is above this line and depressed when it is below this line.

For a discussion of the causes of abnormal ST segments, see Section 2, page 77.

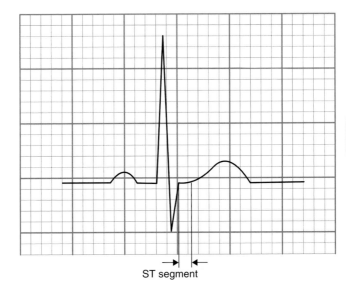

ST segment

12. T wave

In a normal ECG the T wave in most leads is the first deflection from the baseline occurring after the QRS complex. It is caused by ventricular repolarisation.

What is normal?

T waves should be upright in all leads except aVR, III, aVL and V1 where it can be normal to have *isolated* T wave inversion. In the limb leads, the T wave is usually greatest in amplitude in lead II, where up to 6 mm is regarded as normal. In the chest leads it is usually highest in V3, where it can be normal to have a T wave up to 12 mm in height.

CLINICAL TIP

T waves often have subtle abnormalities and a number of possible causes for those abnormalities. The history is vital in helping to determine the likely cause of T wave changes on an ECG. A rule of thumb to use with T waves is—the deeper the inversion, the more likely it is to be a pathological cause.

For a discussion of abnormal T waves, see Section 2, page 86.

13. QT interval

The QT interval is measured from the onset of the QRS complex to the return of the T wave to baseline. It represents the interval from onset of ventricular depolarisation to the offset of ventricular repolarisation.

What is normal?

The QT interval varies with the heart rate. The faster the heart rate, the faster depolarisation/repolarisation occurs, giving a smaller value for the QT interval. To correct for variation due to heart rate, the corrected QT (QTc) is used.

The normal QTc is < 0.45 seconds.

Calculating QTc

The formula most used is Bazett's formula.

$$QTc = \frac{QT(seconds)}{\sqrt{R \text{ to } R \text{ interval}(seconds)}}$$

All measurements are in seconds. These intervals are best measured using the ECG ruler on the back cover of this book.

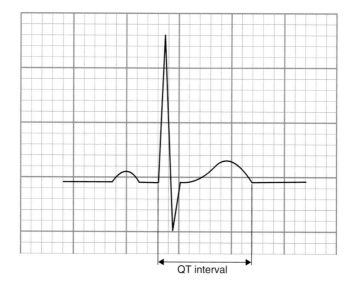

QT interval

> **CLINICAL TIP**
>
> A rule of thumb is that the QT interval should be less than half the interval between two R waves.

 For a discussion of abnormal QTc intervals, see Section 2, page 88.

1

14. Frontal plane axis

The electrical axis is the sum of the electrical vectors during depolarisation. The term 'axis' usually refers to the QRS axis as measured in the limb leads. The electrical axis can also be calculated for P waves and T waves.

How is it calculated?

The height of the QRS signal in two of the limb leads (I, II, III) is measured and plotted on the graph on page 32. A line is drawn at right angles from the end of this line. From this intersection point a line is drawn back to the origin of the graph and the angle of this line from the abscissa is the electrical axis.

What is normal?

The normal QRS axis is between −30 and +105 degrees.

> **CLINICAL TIP**
>
> Calculating the exact value of the axis is an interesting academic exercise but of little clinical value. Hence, broad categories are used clinically—left or right axis deviation, normal axis and indeterminate axis. With practice, one recognises the axis category quickly and easily on the ECG.

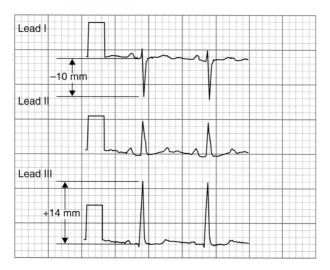

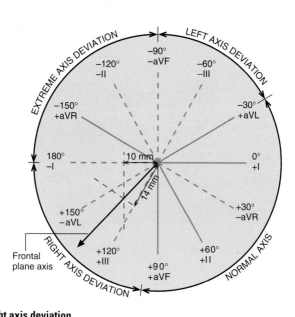

Right axis deviation

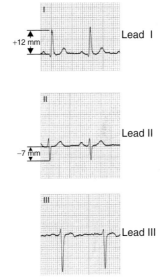

Lead I

Lead II

Lead III

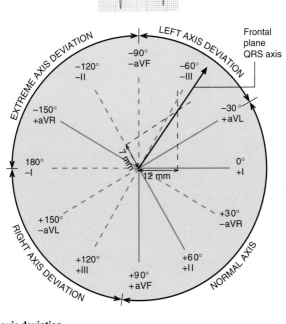

Left axis deviation

SECTION 2

COMMON ABNORMALITIES

When going through the diagnostic steps for an ECG, the clinician often sees something that he/she thinks is abnormal. One of the most difficult steps in ECG interpretation is to diagnose these abnormalities accurately and then place them correctly in the overall context of the ECG and clinical jigsaw.

This section of the handbook is to help you diagnose abnormalities that may have become obvious during the stepwise interpretation undertaken in Section 1.

You will note that this section is set out in the same sequence, reinforcing the recommended sequence for interpreting an ECG and allowing easy reference between the two sections during interpretation. As you work through an ECG, use this method, noting possible differential diagnoses. Once you reach the end of this process you will have a list of ECG diagnoses that can then be interpreted in clinical context.

Section 2 is also a reference for definitions of many common abnormalities and it will help you uncover the importance of each of these abnormalities in reaching an accurate and thorough diagnosis.

HEART RATE

The heart rate is divided into a tachycardia, bradycardia or normal. The category into which the patient's rate falls guides us to the abnormalities that may be present. It must be remembered that it can be normal, when resting, to have sinus rhythm that is a bradycardia or sinus rhythm that is a tachycardia during exercise.

Tachycardia
A patient is said to have a tachycardia when the heart rate exceeds 100 beats per minute.

Causes
Arrhythmias are a cause of tachycardia that are commonly sought on the ECG. These include atrial fibrillation, atrial flutter, supraventricular tachycardia and ventricular tachycardia.

Sinus tachycardia is the most common explanation for a fast heart rate. The causes of this can be divided into normal physiological responses such as exercise, pain or emotional distress and abnormal conditions such as thyrotoxicosis, sepsis, pulmonary embolism, hypovolaemia or heart failure.

Sinus tachycardia occurs when a stimulus is driving the sinus node to depolarise at a faster rate. Catecholamines from exercise or physiological stress are the commonest stimulus.

CLINICAL TIP

Sinus tachycardia in a patient at rest is a sign of physiological stress. It may be the only sign of a serious underlying condition and the cause should be sought immediately.

2

Bradycardia

Bradycardia is arbitrarily defined as a heart rate less than 60 beats per minute.

Causes

It is normal to have a bradycardia at rest, especially while deeply asleep. Trained athletes can have sinus bradycardias even with mild exertion.

Cardiac conduction system disease can lead to bradycardia either by disease or failure of the sinus node or complete block to conduction via the atrioventricular node. Systemic causes of a sinus bradycardia include drugs such as beta-blockers and vagal response to stress which occurs in fainting, hypothyroidism and hypothermia.

Normal

The normal heart rate when resting is 60–100 beats per minute.

RHYTHM

For the purposes of triaging heart rhythms into diagnostic categories we divide the rhythm of the QRS complexes into regular, regular with occasional irregular beats or totally irregular rhythms. Each category carries with it diagnostic implications and, in most cases, the combination of rhythm category and QRS width gives us a good guide to the underlying rhythm.

Regular rhythms

A regular rhythm is one where the timing of each beat is very similar. It is normal to see some minor variation in heart rate with respiration

Sinus tachycardia

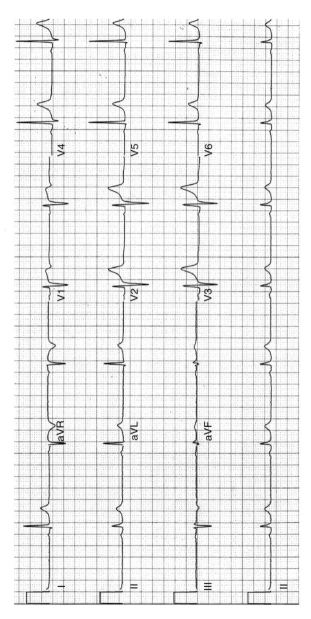

Sinus bradycardia

(sinus arrhythmia), especially in children and young adults. Regular rhythms may arise because of regular spontaneous discharge of pacemaker cells (automatic rhythm), or because of re-entry of a wavefront of excitation around an electrical circuit within the heart (re-entrant arrhythmia).

Sinus rhythm

This is the normal cardiac rhythm; depolarisation originates in the sinoatrial node, which is situated in the high right atrium. This depolarisation spreads through the atrial muscle to the atrioventricular node and after a short delay is conducted to the ventricular conducting system.

Diagnostic features

There is a P wave preceding all QRS complexes; the P waves are normal in axis, being upright in I, II, aVF and V3 to V6. It is normal for the P wave to be inverted in aVR. The P wave is seen prior to each QRS in normal sinus rhythm and the rate of the P waves is the same as the QRS rate. There is a fixed interval on all beats between the P wave and the following QRS complex.

Variations

Sinus arrhythmia is diagnosed when the P-P interval (and consequent heart rate) varies with respiration. It gradually increases with inspiration and decreases with expiration. This is more prevalent in young people and is usually normal.

When the rate is < 60 per minute sinus rhythm is referred to as sinus bradycardia, and when the rate is > 100 it is called a sinus tachycardia.

CLINICAL TIP

Sinus arrhythmia is common in younger people, the incidence decreasing as the age of the patient increases.

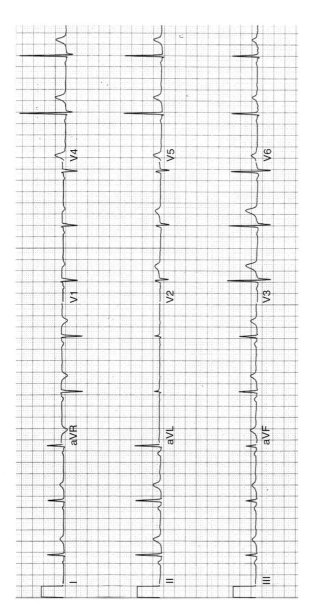

Normal sinus rhythm

Ventricular tachycardia

This is a regular broad complex tachycardia. The QRS complexes are over three small squares (> 0.12 s) in width.

Ventricular tachycardia is usually caused by a short circuit in the ventricular muscle at the edge of a scar. The ventricle is controlled by this short circuit and it in turn controls all electrical activation of the heart.

Diagnostic features

Ventricular tachycardia has broad QRS complexes without preceding P waves. Rarely P waves may be seen but they have no fixed relationship to the QRS complexes unless there is 1:1 conduction back to the atrium via the atrioventricular node. If this is occurring the P waves are seen after the QRS complex, in the T wave.

Variations

All regular broad QRS complex tachycardias should be regarded as ventricular tachycardia as this is the most dangerous cause of this pattern. Differential diagnoses include supraventricular tachycardia or sinus tachycardia with conduction across the atrioventricular junction via an accessory pathway or a ventricular bundle branch block.

CLINICAL TIP

All patients with a regular broad complex tachycardia should be regarded as having ventricular tachycardia. Resuscitation must be immediately available. This is because of the propensity of this arrhythmia to degenerate to the potentially fatal ventricular fibrillation. It is better to overtreat a supraventricular tachycardia with bundle branch block than to undertreat a case of ventricular tachycardia.

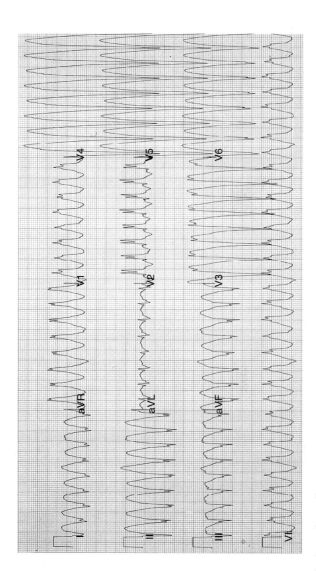

Ventricular tachycardia

Atrial flutter

This is an atrial re-entrant tachycardia in which the atria usually depolarise at 300 beats per minute. The ventricular rate is determined by the amount of block to conduction provided by the atrioventricular node. In untreated cases the resulting ventricular rate is usually a factor of 300 (i.e. 2:1 atrioventricular block gives a rate of 150 bpm, 3:1 gives 100 bpm etc.). The commonest is 2:1 atrioventricular block giving a QRS rate of 150 bpm.

The commonest atrial flutter comes from the right atrium. There is an abnormal circuit that circles around the right atrium with a critical isthmus between the tricuspid valve and the inferior vena cava. The atria depolarise in a coordinated manner at 300 per minute giving the characteristic flutter waves on the ECG.

Diagnostic features

In most cases of atrial flutter the rapid and abnormally shaped P waves occur at a rate of 300 per minute (one per large grid square—0.20 s). The appearance is commonly referred to as 'saw-tooth' because the shape of the P waves is similar to that of the teeth on a wood saw.

A patient can have both atrial flutter and atrial fibrillation. The flutter occurs in the right atrium and simultaneously the left atrium can fibrillate. On the ECG the saw-tooth appearance is usually seen in lead V1, but the rhythm is irregularly irregular in timing. This is often reported as atrial flutter/fibrillation.

CLINICAL TIP

Occasionally, a tachycardia will be seen with a QRS rate of 150 bpm and no obvious P waves. A manoeuvre to increase atrioventricular block, such as forced expiration against a closed glottis (Valsalva technique), may slow atrioventricular conduction and reduce ventricular rate, thereby revealing the flutter waves. This tells us atrial flutter is the cause of tachycardia, rather than a re-entrant supraventricular tachycardia with anterograde conduction via the atrioventricular node and retrograde conduction via an accessory pathway.

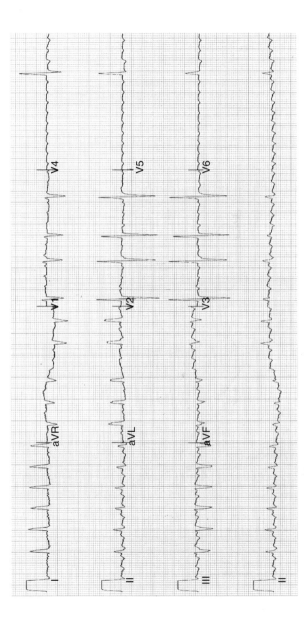

Atrial flutter during the Valsalva manoeuvre

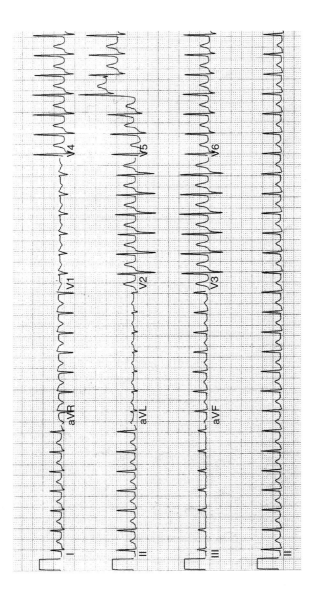

Supraventricular tachycardia (SVT)

Supraventricular tachycardia

Supraventricular tachycardia (SVT) is a confusing term. While its literal interpretation means tachycardias above the ventricle, in clinical practice the term SVT has come to be used exclusively for arrhythmias that utilise the atrioventricular node and an accessory connection (or short circuit) for their re-entrant circuit. They can travel either from atria to ventricle via the AV node and return to the atria via the accessory connection (known as orthodromic) or vice versa (antidromic). The best known condition that predisposes to SVT is the Wolff-Parkinson-White syndrome.

> *People who experience SVT are born with extra muscle strands across the fibrous atrioventricular junction. These fibres conduct electrical impulses. If they conduct from atrium to ventricle, the ECG shows Wolff-Parkinson-White pattern. Some fibres only conduct from the ventricle to the atrium and are not seen on the ECG. SVT occurs when there is electricity travelling one direction in the muscle fibres and the other way through the AV node. This sets up the re-entry circuit needed to sustain SVT.*

Diagnostic features

Classically, SVT is a narrow QRS complex regular tachycardia. The rate of the tachycardia is usually 170–260 bpm and is constant at this tachycardia heart rate. If the tachycardia is due to an accessory pathway (the commonest being Wolff-Parkinson-White syndrome) then retrograde P waves are often visible between the QRS complexes.

When SVT is due to atrioventricular nodal re-entry tachycardia, retrograde P waves are not visible as they coincide with the QRS complex.

In rare cases, SVT can cause a wide complex tachycardia on the ECG. This occurs when the tachycardia travels from atria to ventricle via the accessory connection (antidromic) or when there is a rate-related block to conduction in one of the bundle branches during tachycardia. Unless the patient is known to have one of these two phenomena, all wide complex tachycardias are best regarded as ventricular tachycardia (VT) and treated as such, because the ECG criteria for differentiating SVT with broad QRS and VT are not sufficiently specific nor sensitive to rely on in the clinical situation.

CLINICAL TIP

If a patient with a broad complex tachycardia is haemo-dynamically stable, manoeuvres such as forced expiration against a closed glottis (the Valsalva technique), carotid sinus massage or drugs that block the atrioventricular node such as adenosine may be used, while recording an ECG as a diagnostic technique. This should only be done in a high-dependency resuscitation area.

In the patient has ventricular tachycardia it will remain unaffected, a transient increase in atrioventricular block may occur in atrial flutter revealing saw-tooth flutter waves, and SVT will often revert to sinus rhythm.

In the elderly, carotid sinus massage should be used with extreme caution because of the risk of dislodging plaque from the carotid artery.

AV junctional escape rhythm

This is a rhythm where the origin of cardiac depolarisation is in the atrioventricular junction. An escape rhythm occurs when there is failure of the sinus node to depolarise and maintain normal sinus rhythm.

Diagnostic features

The QRS complexes occur without a preceding P wave. The QRS complexes are often slightly wider than normal (2–3 small squares, 0.08–0.12 s) and occasionally a retrograde (upside-down) P wave can be seen after each QRS complex, usually embedded in the T wave. This P wave is usually a result of retrograde activation of the atrium from the junctional region. The rate of a junctional escape rhythm is usually between 40 and 60 per minute.

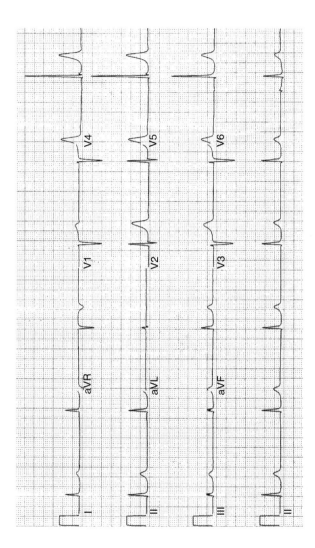

Junctional rhythm

Regular rhythms with occasional irregular beats

Sinus rhythm with atrial ectopic beats

This is a sinus rhythm with early narrow complex beats from an atrial or pulmonary vein focus.

Diagnostic features

These premature beats may or may not have a P wave preceding them. This is because often the P wave occurs quite early and is disguised on the ECG within the T wave from the preceding beat. The resultant QRS from an atrial ectopic beat is of narrow complex (unlike ventricular ectopic beats). The beat occurs before the next sinus beat is due and resets the sinus node so that the next sinus beat occurs later than would have been the case in the absence of the ectopic beat.

If the P wave from the atrial ectopic is visible, it will have a different morphology and axis from normal P waves.

Variations

If the atrial ectopic beats are frequent they can make the rhythm appear irregular. With close inspection one can see that the underlying rhythm is still sinus node in origin and the early beats are ectopics.

> CLINICAL TIP
>
> Extremely frequent atrial ectopic beats may be a predisposing factor to developing atrial fibrillation. There are some patients with ectopic foci situated in their pulmonary veins who also experience paroxysmal atrial fibrillation. If the patient has symptoms of more sustained irregular palpitations this should be investigated further.

Sinus rhythm with ventricular ectopic beats

This is a sinus rhythm with early beats from a ventricular focus.

Diagnostic features

The premature beats have wide QRS complexes (greater than three small squares, > 0.12 s). If they occur paired with each sinus beat it is referred to as *bigeminy*.

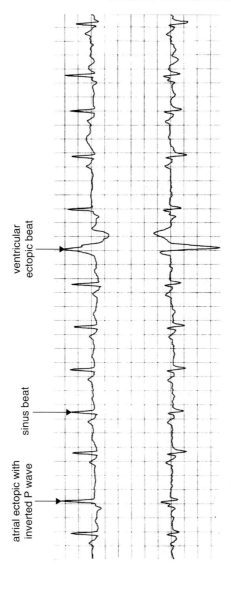

Sinus rhythm with atrial and ventricular beats

> **CLINICAL TIP**
> Ventricular ectopic beats are more frequent during periods of fatigue, stress or excess consumption of stimulants such as caffeine. They may also occur frequently during pregnancy and menopause.

Irregular rhythms

Atrial fibrillation

This is a totally irregular or apparently random rhythm with no evidence of discrete P waves preceding each (usually narrow) QRS complex. This pattern is referred to as 'irregularly irregular'.

> *In atrial fibrillation, there are multiple short circuits in the atrial muscle. These are started by either an abnormality in the atrial muscle or from ectopic foci in the pulmonary veins. These multiple low voltage short circuits are seen either as fine low amplitude 'f' waves or no atrial electrical activity.*

Diagnostic features

Atrial fibrillation is an 'irregularly irregular' rhythm with no rhythm or regular 'beat' to the QRS complexes. Small fine fibrillation impulses (or 'f' waves) may be seen between the QRS complexes.

Variations

Atrial fibrillation can occur in the left atrium while atrial flutter is occurring in the right atrium. In this situation you may see some organisation to the atrial activity in the form of flutter waves at times, usually in lead V1, while the rest of the atrial rhythm is composed of 'f' waves. The ventricular (QRS) rate is determined by the rate of conduction through the AV node. If the ventricular rate is a tachycardia, the atrial fibrillation is said to be uncontrolled.

> **CLINICAL TIP**
> During atrial fibrillation there are no P waves on the ECG, hence you cannot offer a comment on the size of the atria in your ECG interpretation.

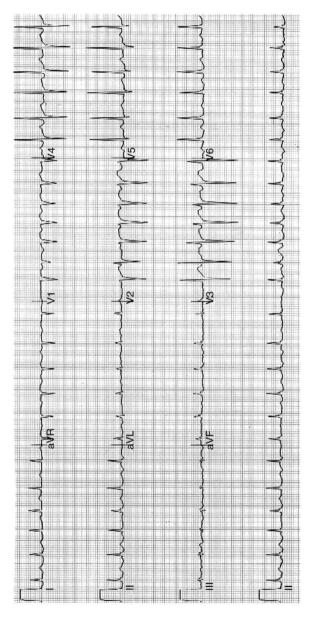

Atrial fibrillation

Ventricular fibrillation

This shows fine rapid irregular low-amplitude electrical activity. There is no discreet QRS complex and no cardiac output. This is a fatal condition unless treated rapidly. The patient will be unrousable and have no pulse.

> ### CLINICAL TIP
>
> Ventricular fibrillation is a fatal condition unless treated rapidly by DC cardioversion. The sooner after the onset of ventricular fibrillation the DC shock is delivered, the greater the chance of resuscitation. Cardiopulmonary resuscitation should be instituted if there is a delay in the arrival of a defibrillator.

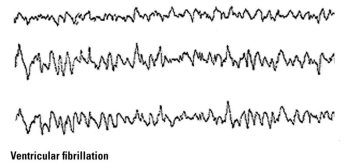

Ventricular fibrillation

P WAVES

Changes from the normal P wave give us a guide to the underlying atrial chamber size. You can only measure P waves and offer comment on atrial chamber size when the patient is in sinus rhythm.

P pulmonale
Peaked P waves > 2.5 mm (which is > 2.5 mV) in height in leads II, III and aVF plus a biphasic P wave in V1, with the initial upwards deflection greater than the following negative deflection. The duration of the P waves is usually normal (< 0.12 s).

Cause
P pulmonale is caused by right atrial hypertrophy and, as the name suggests, is most commonly seen in patients with lung disease causing secondary pulmonary hypertension.

In right atrial hypertrophy there is more atrial muscle mass and hence higher voltages. This is reflected as taller P waves.

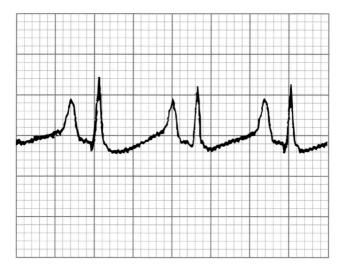

Tall P waves of right atrial hypertrophy

P mitrale

P waves of abnormally long duration (> 0.11 s) in any lead. The P wave may have an obvious double hump, or M shape. The first hump represents right atrial depolarisation, the second hump being the depolarisation of the enlarged left atrium. The amplitude is usually normal (< 2.5 mm).

Cause

P mitrale is caused by left atrial dilation. Enlargement of the left atrium is often due to mitral valve disease, hence the name of the ECG finding, P mitrale.

As the left atrium dilates, it takes longer for the depolarisation to spread. Right atrial depolarisation is completed quickly and is seen as the first hump on the M shaped P wave. The second hump is the completion of the delayed left atrial depolarisation.

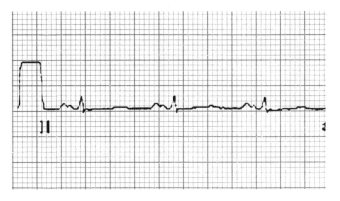

Wide P waves of left atrial enlargement

PR INTERVAL

When assessing the PR interval, remember that it is measured from the start of the P wave to the start of the QRS complex. It is a common mistake to measure from the end of the P wave to the start of the QRS complex.

It is a measure of the time for conduction from the sinus node to the first ventricular activation. The duration of this interval is mostly determined by the time taken for the depolarisation wavefront to cross the atrioventricular junction.

> **CLINICAL TIP**
> As with any interval on the ECG, if the PR interval is very abnormal check the calibration signal on the ECG—incorrect ECG paper speed will give an incorrect interval measurement.

Short PR interval
PR interval < 0.12 seconds.

The normal PR interval is due primarily to the delay in conduction through the atrioventricular node. Shortening of this interval indicates that either the electrical impulse is getting through the atrioventricular junction quicker than normal, or that the origin of the impulse is coming from close to the atrioventricular node.

Causes
- **Wolff-Parkinson-White syndrome (WPW).** Check for slurring of the upstroke of the QRS complex (delta wave). This in combination with a short PR is diagnostic of this condition. Rapid conduction of the depolarisation wavefront via an accessory pathway (short circuit) from atrium to ventricle during sinus rhythm gives us the characteristic findings of Wolff-Parkinson-White syndrome. With WPW you will often notice the PR interval is shorter and the delta wave is more pronounced in some leads. This is a normal feature of WPW and can be a guide to determining where in the heart the accessory pathway lies. Occasionally, repolarisation abnormalities are seen as ST changes.

Wolff-Parkinson-White syndrome

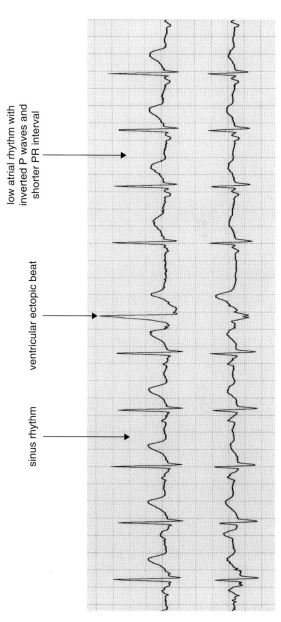

low atrial rhythm with inverted P waves and shorter PR interval

ventricular ectopic beat

sinus rhythm

WPW predisposes to supraventricular tachycardia during which the wavefront of excitation usually passes retrogradely over the accessory pathway from ventricle to atrium, and then returns from the atrium to ventricle via the normal atrioventricular node.

An uncommon variant in patients with an accessory pathway is where the tachycardia passes in the opposite direction, from atrium to ventricle via the accessory pathway, and from ventricle to atrium via the atrioventricular node. This results in a broad complex tachycardia.

CLINICAL TIP

The accessory pathway in Wolff-Parkinson-White syndrome may conduct atrial fibrillation to the ventricle without delay, leading to ventricular fibrillation and sudden death. All patients with WPW should be considered for ablation of their accessory pathway.

- **Lown-Ganong-Levine syndrome.** Causes a short PR interval with normal QRS (no delta wave).
- **Ectopic pacemaker.** If there is an ectopic atrial pacemaker situated low in the atrium near the AV node the conduction time of this impulse to the AV node (and hence the PR interval) is shortened. This is diagnosed by an abnormal P wave axis in conjunction with the short PR interval.

Long PR interval

PR interval > 5 small squares (> 0.20 s).

Lengthening of the PR interval is caused by delay in conduction through the atrioventricular node. The amount of delay and the pattern of this delay gives us a classification scheme for describing the ECG abnormality. The underlying causes for lengthening of the PR interval are not reflected in the classification below, and should be sought in each case of atrioventricular conduction delay.

Diagnoses

- **First-degree atrioventricular block.** The PR interval is > 5 small squares (> 0.20 s) and there is a constant relationship between the P and R waves. All atrial impulses are conducted to the ventricle albeit with the prolonged PR interval.
- **Second-degree atrioventricular block.** This is diagnosed when there is intermittent failure of the P waves to be conducted to the ventricle.

In Mobitz type 1 or Wenckebach phenomenon there is progressive lengthening of the PR interval until a P wave is not conducted. This results in intermittent dropping of a QRS complex in the rhythm.

In Mobitz type 2 there is a constant PR interval (normal or prolonged) with intermittent failure of conduction of a P wave to the ventricle.

CLINICAL TIP

It is common for patients to have transient second-degree atrioventricular block or for them to alternate between Mobitz type 1 and Mobitz type 2 block.

- **Third-degree atrioventricular block.** This is diagnosed when there is no regular relationship of the P waves to the QRS complexes. In this condition there is complete AV conduction block. A ventricular pacemaker site generates the QRS complexes. Usually this is high in the ventricle but, in older patients and in those with more diffusely diseased hearts, the escape complex may come from a low ventricular site. Generally, the lower in the ventricle the escape pacemaker is situated, the wider the QRS complex and the slower the QRS rate.

  Occasionally, patients do not generate a ventricular escape rhythm and, in this circumstance, when complete heart block occurs it may be a terminal event.

As the AV node becomes diseased, it takes longer to repolarise and becomes slower in the speed of conduction. This is reflected initially as a prolonged PR interval and subsequently as higher degree block.

P wave   QRS

prolonged
PR interval

First-degree atrioventricular block

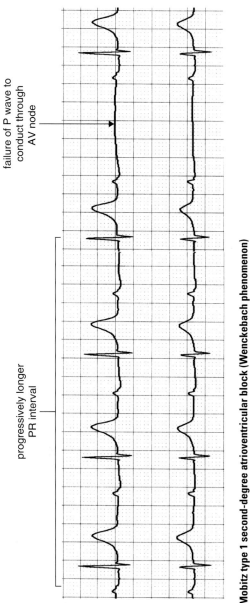

failure of P wave to conduct through AV node

progressively longer PR interval

Mobitz type 1 second-degree atrioventricular block (Wenckebach phenomenon)

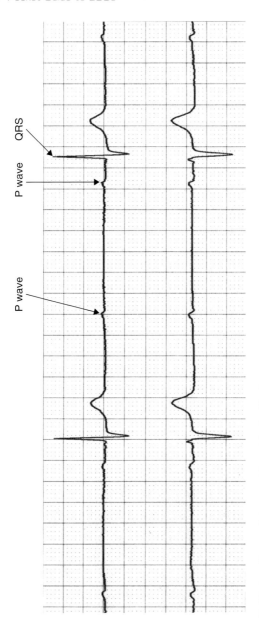

Mobitz type 2 second-degree atrioventricular block

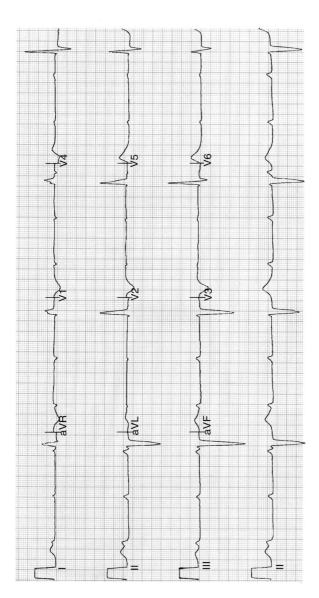

Third-degree complete atrioventricular block

QRS COMPLEX DURATION PROLONGED

QRS duration is prolonged when it is more than 3 small squares in width (> 0.12 s).

Causes
There are two common causes for QRS prolongation.

1. Disease in the ventricular part of the conduction system such as in the bundle branches beyond the bundle of His. The rhythm, originating from the atrium or less commonly the junctional region, is delayed in conduction through the ventricular conduction system, showing as a widened QRS complex on ECG.
2. The second and less common cause of a widened QRS complex is a rhythm originating in the ventricle.

There are three causes of this: the most dangerous is ventricular tachycardia. The slower ventricular (idioventricular) escape rhythm seen in complete heart block gives a wide QRS and, as mentioned previously, the lower its origin in the ventricle the wider the complex. The third, increasingly common, cause is ventricular pacing. With increased availability of implanted pacemakers there are more people with a pacing spike on the ECG prior to the QRS complex.

The conducting system in the ventricle allows fast transit of the depolarisation after it exits the atrioventricular node. When part of the ventricular conduction system is diseased the depolarisation wavefront must take the slower route, via the myocardium. This results in the wider intervals we notice on the ECG.

Diagnoses
If the rhythm has P waves preceding each complex, or the rhythm is irregularly irregular (atrial fibrillation), there are four possible diagnoses for the prolonged ventricular conduction.

Right bundle branch block (RBBB)
This is diagnosed when the QRS is > 3 small squares (0.12 s) with an rSR (M-shaped) positive QRS in V1 and/or a W-shaped negative complex in V6.

Right bundle branch block, as the name suggests, is due to complete block of conduction down the right bundle branch beyond the bundle of His. The right ventricle is therefore depolarised by the wave of activation spreading through the ventricular myocardium from the left ventricle (which has been swiftly activated by conduction down the left bundle branch). Depolarisation via the myocardium is slower than via the normal bundle branch and hence the QRS complex is wider than normal.

Bifascicular block is the term used to describe the presence of complete right bundle branch block with left anterior fascicular block, or the more uncommon combination of complete right bundle branch block with left posterior fascicular block.

Partial right bundle branch block
This is diagnosed when the QRS duration is 0.10–0.12 seconds in duration and V1 and/or V6 has the morphology of RBBB.

Left bundle branch block (LBBB)
This is diagnosed when the QRS is > 3 small squares (0.12 s) with a W-shaped negative complex in V1 and/or a positive M-shaped complex in V6. This is caused by complete conduction block in the left branch of the bundle of His. The left ventricle is thus activated from the conduction via the myocardium spreading from the right ventricle.

CLINICAL TIP

The diagnosis of complete left bundle branch block in the presence of a clinical history and physical signs of myocardial infarction should be treated as a myocardial infarction. The bundle branch block makes the ST segments uninterpretable, and large clinical trials have shown that reperfusion therapy should be instituted in this setting as it confers a survival benefit.

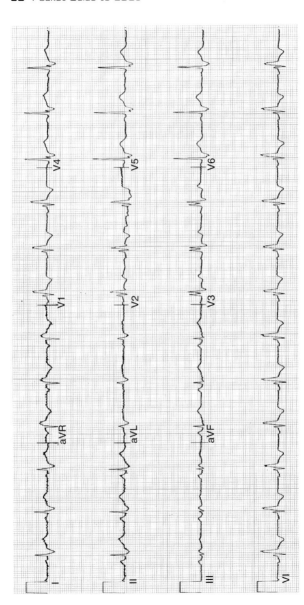

Sinus rhythm with right bundle branch block

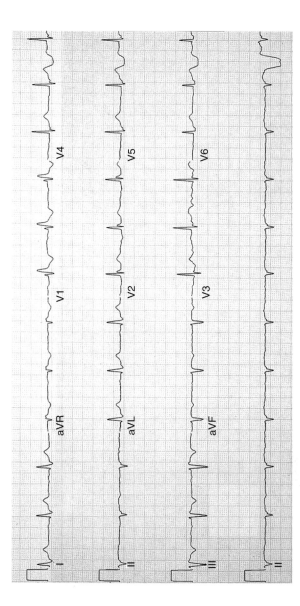

Sinus rhythm with bifascicular block (RBBB + left anterior fascicular block)

Sinus rhythm with partial right bundle branch block

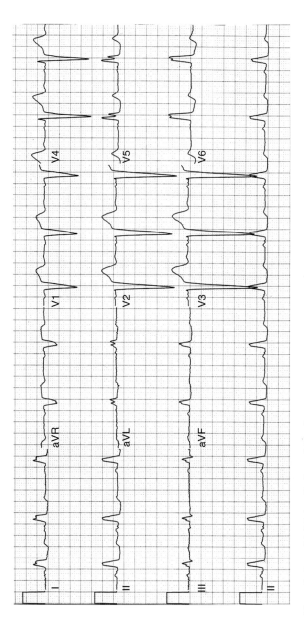

Sinus rhythm with left bundle branch block

Intraventricular conduction delay

This is diagnosed when the QRS duration is 0.10–0.12 seconds and the QRS morphology is not typical LBBB or RBBB pattern.

Rule of thumb for bundle branch block patterns

When the QRS is prolonged and you are trying to remember which bundle branch is blocked, ask William Morrow.

Shape in V1	Bundle branch affected	Shape in V6
W	i LL ia	M
M	o RR o	W

Other causes of a wide QRS complex

Ventricular tachycardia

If the rhythm is a regular tachycardia without P waves preceding each QRS, the diagnosis should be regarded as ventricular tachycardia and the patient treated accordingly.

> CLINICAL TIP
>
> The diagnosis of ventricular tachycardia is more likely if the patient has a history of myocardial infarction or structural heart disease. The more extensive the damage from the infarction the more likely the patient is to have ventricular tachycardia. The absence of structural heart disease does not exclude ventricular tachycardia; it does, however, make it less likely.

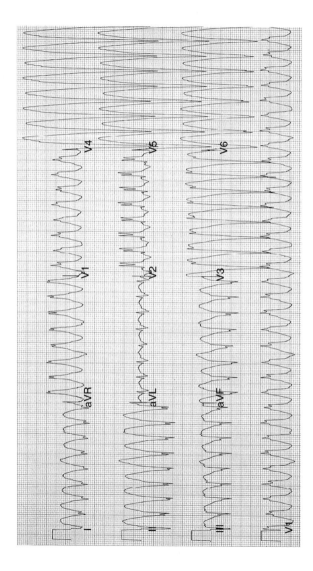

Ventricular tachycardia

Ventricular escape rhythm

If the rhythm is regular and slow (< 60 per minute) and there are no regular P waves preceding the QRS, consider a ventricular escape rhythm as occurs in complete atrioventricular block (third-degree heart block).

Pacemaker

If the patient has a pacemaker and the QRS under scrutiny is caused by an impulse from the pacemaker, you will often see a small sharp pacing spike at the commencement of the QRS. Older unipolar pacemakers have large obvious pacing spikes before the device-stimulated complexes. Bipolar pacemakers, which are now the standard type used, have only small spikes and one must consider paced rhythm as an option when the QRS is of left bundle branch block morphology.

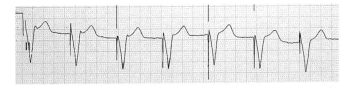

Ventricular pacing

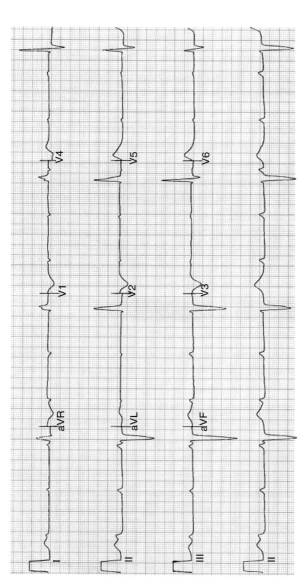

Complete atrioventricular block with a slow ventricular escape rhythm

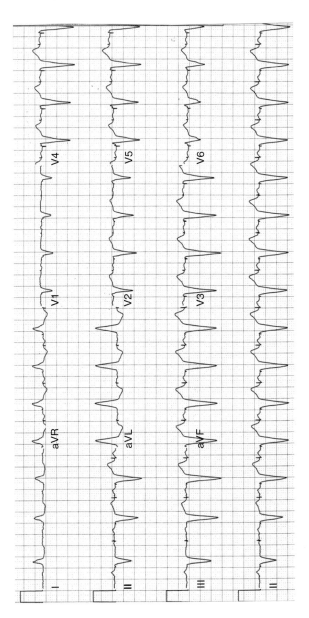

Dual chamber (atrial and ventricular) pacing

ST SEGMENTS ABNORMAL

The ST segments are abnormal if they are elevated or depressed > 1 mm from the isoelectric line.

> **CLINICAL TIP**
>
> ST segment abnormalities can only be interpreted adequately in the context of a clinical history. While there are some 'classic' patterns to ST elevation and depression, these are neither specific nor sensitive enough to preclude the need for a clinical history and examination.

ST elevation

Transmural myocardial infarction

Classically, this has an arched appearance (convex upwards) with the ST segment being upsloping rather than the normal horizontal ST segment. The area over which the ST elevation occurs indicates the part of the heart that is infarcting. Any ST elevation, in the presence of history and examination findings consistent with myocardial infarction, should be treated as such. ST elevation > 1 mm in leads II, III and aVF indicates inferior myocardial infarction; elevation of the ST segment > 2 mm in V1 to V4 indicates anterior wall infarction; if this extends to V5 and V6, it is anterolateral wall infarction. ST elevation in the 'high lateral' leads I and aVL often accompanies anterolateral infarction.

Area of heart affected	Leads with ST elevation
Inferior wall	II, III, aVF
Anterior wall	V1 to V4
Lateral wall	V5, V6 and occasionally I and aVL
Posterior wall	ST depression in V1 to V3

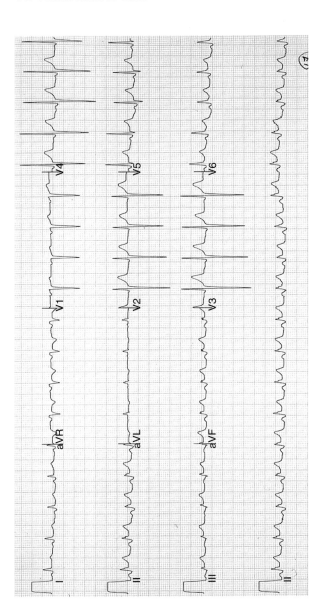

Sinus rhythm with acute inferior infarction

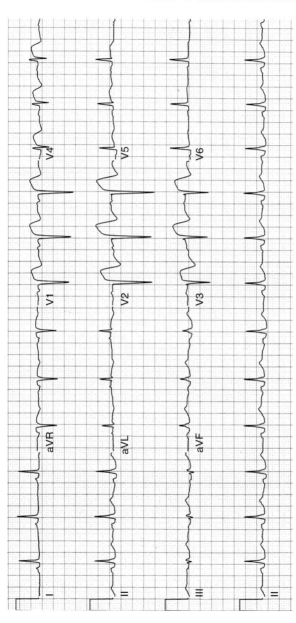

Sinus rhythm with acute anterior infarction

> **CLINICAL TIP**
> Inferior wall acute infarction requires only 1 mm of ST elevation for the diagnosis, whereas anterior and anterolateral acute infarction require 2 mm.

Early repolarisation

So-called early repolarisation pattern ST elevation is sometimes seen in young people and is more common in African and African American people. It is characterised by elevation of the J point and concave upwards-type ST elevation.

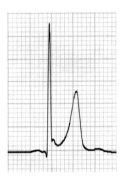

Early repolarisation type ST elevation

Ventricular aneurysm

ST elevation persisting for longer than one week after a myocardial infarction raises the possibility of ventricular aneurysm formation. If the ST elevation is still present at one month after infarction, it is most likely due to ventricular aneurysm formation. The ST elevation is usually preceded by deep Q waves of transmural infarction. There is associated loss of the R waves and occasionally T wave inversion.

Pericarditis

Pericarditis is difficult to diagnose confidently on ECG criteria alone. Usually, the ST elevation is horizontal or concave upward, and widespread throughout all leads, although in some cases it can be localised. There is usually still a distinction between the ST segment and T wave and it may be accompanied by depression of the PR segment.

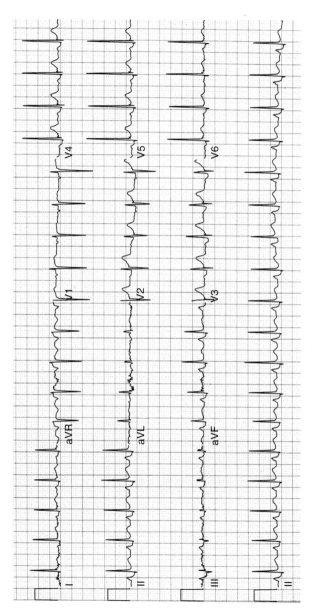

Sinus rhythm with PR segment depression and ST elevation consistent with pericarditis

CLINICAL TIP

Pericarditis is often a diagnosis made after myocardial infarction has been excluded. As with many ECG diagnoses, the clinical history assumes greater importance than the nuances of the ST elevation in distinguishing pericarditis from myocardial infarction.

Vasospastic angina

Vasospastic angina, also known as Prinzmetal's angina, causes ST segment elevation during the chest pain that mimics transmural myocardial infarction. The ST segments return to normal once the chest pain is relieved. On a resting ECG with no history one cannot differentiate between Prinzmetal's angina and myocardial infarction; hence this variant of angina is a diagnosis made on a combination of history and ECG findings.

ST SEGMENT DEPRESSION

Ischaemia is the first diagnosis that should come to mind when ST depression is seen. If the patient has symptoms that may be due to myocardial ischaemia—even if other ECG causes for the ST segment changes are present—the patient should initially be regarded as having myocardial ischaemia.

Ischaemia

Depression of the ST segments, particularly if occurring during chest pain, is highly suggestive of myocardial ischaemia. Ischaemic ST depression is often horizontal or downsloping, meaning that the J point is ≥ 1 mm (0.1 mV) below the isoelectric line, and the ST segments are horizontal or downwards sloping. It is accompanied usually by T wave inversion.

CLINICAL TIP

ST depression occurring during exercise or during episodes of chest pain should be regarded as due to myocardial ischaemia. The deeper the ST depression that occurs with exercise, the more significant the ischaemia.

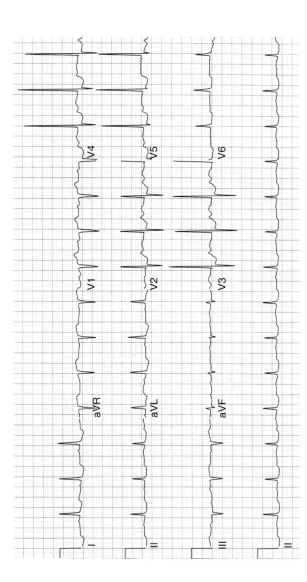

Sinus rhythm with anterolateral ischaemia

Left ventricular hypertrophy

ST depression is a common finding in people with ECG voltage criteria for left ventricular hypertrophy. It is seen in leads V5 and V6 and is downwards sloping and accompanied by T wave inversion.

Left ventricular hypertrophy is diagnosed on an ECG based on the size of the voltages in the QRS complexes. If the R wave in V6 + the S wave in V2 is > 35 mm, or the R wave in V5 + the S wave in V1 is > 35 mm, or the voltage in any of leads I, II or III is > 20 mm, then LVH is diagnosed by voltage criteria.

CLINICAL TIP

When voltage criteria for LVH are met, check the ECG calibration signal to ensure it is correct. The diagnosis of LVH should be confirmed by another modality, as the voltage in the chest leads also depends on the distance from the heart at which the electrodes lie. A patient with a very thin chest (such as a child) may have high voltages but a normal left ventricle. Conversely, in a patient who is morbidly obese or has a lung disease and a barrel-shaped chest, normal QRS voltages do not allow confident exclusion of left ventricular hypertrophy.

Digitalis

In some patients digitalis can cause ST depression in leads V5 and V6.

Hypokalaemia

Up to 1 mm of ST depression can occur with low serum potassium levels. T wave flattening and the appearance of prominent U waves and associated widening of the QRS complexes often accompany ST depression as the serum potassium level drops.

Right ventricular hypertrophy

The presence of downsloping ST depression in leads II, III, aVF and V1, V2 is sometimes seen with right ventricular hypertrophy (for full diagnostic criteria, see Section 3).

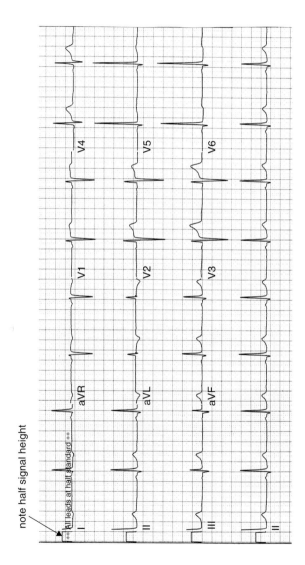

note half signal height

Sinus rhythm with left ventricular hypertrophy NOTE calibration signal

T WAVES ABNORMAL

T waves are regarded as abnormal when they are inverted in leads in which they should be upright, or when they are abnormally tall (see Section 1).

Causes

The T waves may undergo changes in numerous conditions. Changes may be innocent or pathological. An abnormal T wave is often a non-specific finding and its clinical relevance and likely diagnosis can only be made in the context of history and examination of the patient.

Innocent changes
- Juvenile ECG pattern
- Hyperventilation
- Postural change, from lying to standing usually
- Postprandial state
- Young black males
- Trained athletes

Pathological changes
- Hyperacute (very first stages) myocardial infarction (tall peaked T waves in the territory affected)
- Subendocardial (non-transmural) myocardial infarction (deep T wave inversion in contiguous leads)
- Myocardial ischaemia (T wave inversion that resolves when pain resolves)
- Hyperkalaemia (tall, narrow, peaked T waves)
- Hypokalaemia (decreased T wave amplitude)
- Magnesium abnormalities (non-specific T changes)
- Digitalis (decreased amplitude of T wave which may become biphasic or negative).

QT INTERVAL ABNORMAL

The QT interval varies with the heart rate, becoming shorter as the heart rate increases. It is therefore corrected for the heart rate and referred to as the QTc. The QTc should be 450 ms (0.45 seconds) or less in duration to be normal.

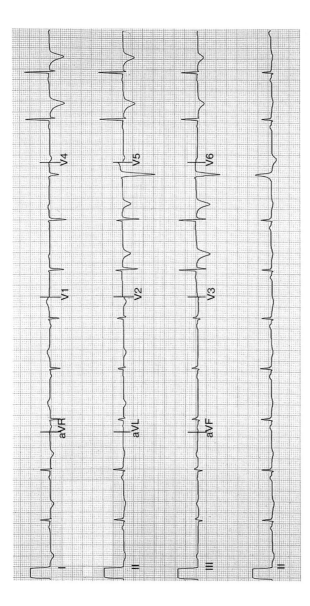

Sinus rhythm with anterolateral subendocardial infarction

Calculation of the QTc

There are several formulae for correcting the measured QT for the heart rate. The most widely used is that of Bazett in which the measured QT interval (in seconds) is divided by the square root of the RR interval (in seconds). The RR interval is the measured interval between two successive R waves on the ECG.

$$QTc = \frac{QT \text{ (seconds)}}{\sqrt{RR \text{ interval (seconds)}}}$$

Rule of thumb for QT

A rule of thumb to use when reviewing an ECG is that the QT interval should be less than half the R to R interval for any two successive complexes. If the QT is equal to, or greater than, half the R to R interval then the QTc should be calculated.

CLINICAL TIP

If there is a clinical history suggestive of QT abnormalities, the QTc must always be calculated. It must also be remembered that the QT interval can vary during a given day or from day to day; hence, in a patient with a history that suggests there may be a QT interval abnormality, consider analysing repeated ECGs or performing prolonged monitoring (Holter monitoring) with QT analysis.

Causes of prolonged QT interval

Drugs

This is not an exhaustive list, but the drugs that more commonly cause QTc prolongation include the antiarrhythmic drugs, some non-sedating antihistamines, erythromycin and psychotropic drugs (especially tricyclic antidepressants and phenothiazines). Any patient who has a prolonged QTc should have a thorough drug history taken and each drug looked up in a pharmacological database to see whether it affects the QT interval.

Idiopathic

A number of idiopathic causes of QT prolongation have been described and the underlying cellular mechanism for some of them has been elucidated. They include Romano-Ward syndrome, Jervell-Lange-Nielson syndrome, Brugada syndrome, and idiopathic long QT syndrome. It is beyond the scope of this text to discuss these conditions in detail.

Metabolic disturbances

These are usually electrolyte disturbances (commonly calcium disorders).

Central nervous system disease

It is common for patients with central nervous system diseases, especially intracranial bleeding, to have ECG abnormalities including QT changes.

DIAGNOSTIC FEATURES OF COMMON DISORDERS (A QUICK REFERENCE)

Often, a number of diagnoses can be made on any given ECG. Patients presenting with a rhythm disorder commonly have a disorder of conduction or concomitant myocardial ischaemia. This section contains an overview of the features of the common disorders diagnosed on ECG. The sequence of interpretation is recommended for the interpretation of all ECGs and follows the sequence of Section 1, pages 16 to 33.

ATRIAL FIBRILLATION

Regular/irregular rhythm	Irregularly irregular, meaning there is random timing to the complexes
P waves present	No; instead you often see fine fibrillation or 'f' waves
Atrial rate	Cannot be measured
QRS rate	Varies depending on drug treatment and AV node conduction time. Usually 100–180 per minute but may be a bradycardia if there is coexisting conduction disease
P and QRS relationship	Not relevant
PR interval	Not relevant
QRS width	Usually narrow complex unless there is a ventricular conduction defect or Wolff-Parkinson-White syndrome; they produce an irregularly irregular broad complex rhythm
ST segments	Non-diagnostic
T waves	Non-diagnostic
Axis	QRS axis is normal in the absence of conducting system disease

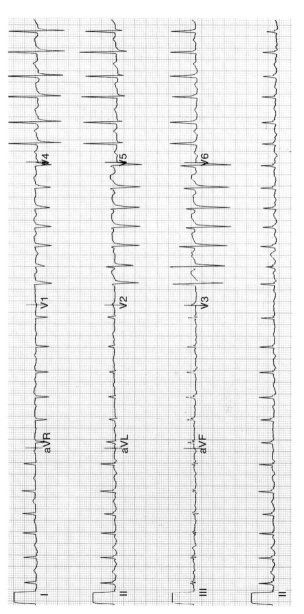

3

Atrial fibrillation

ATRIAL FLUTTER

Regular/irregular rhythm	Regular unless there is varying AV block
P waves present	Yes, 'saw-tooth' P waves are obvious in aVF or V1
Atrial rate	Usually 300 per minute
QRS rate	Classically, it is 150 per minute but depends on the degree of AV block; hence if 3:1 AV block rate will be 300/3 = 100, if 4:1 block rate will be 300/1 = 75 per minute etc.
P and QRS relationship	QRS always preceded by a P wave or multiple P waves; commonly in a fixed pattern, i.e. 2 P waves per QRS in 2:1 AV conduction, 3 P waves per QRS in 3:1 etc.
PR interval	Depends on the degree of AV block
QRS width	Narrow complex unless there is a ventricular conduction defect, in which case you will have an irregularly irregular broad complex rhythm
ST segments	Non-diagnostic
T waves	Non-diagnostic
Axis	QRS axis is normal in the absence of conducting system disease

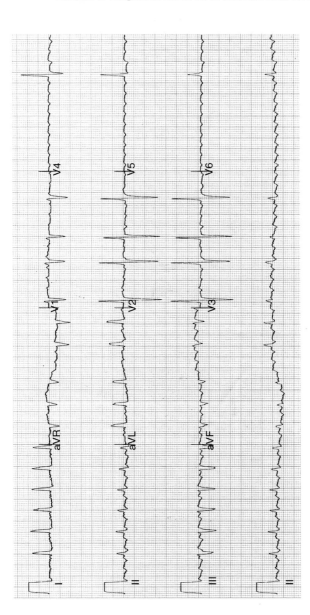

Atrial flutter with increasing atrioventricular block due to Valsalva manoeuvre

3

ATRIAL ECTOPICS

Regular/irregular rhythm	Regular with occasional early QRS if the atrial ectopic is conducted to the ventricle. Atrial bigeminy is when the atrial ectopic beats are paired with sinus beats in a repeating pattern
P waves present	Yes, often inverted and of abnormal morphology on the ectopic beats. Sometimes they are not visible because they fall in the T wave from the preceding beat, in which case we see only an early narrow complex QRS occurring just after the T wave
Atrial rate	The ectopic beat occurs earlier than expected for the next sinus beat
QRS rate	That of the underlying sinus rhythm
P and QRS relationship	Ectopic P may or may not be conducted to the ventricle, depending on how early it occurs and whether the AV node has recovered from the preceding beat
PR interval	Variable, depending on the state of repolarisation of the AV node
QRS width	Usually narrow complex unless there is a ventricular conduction defect
ST segments	Non-diagnostic
T waves	Non-diagnostic
Axis	The P wave axis of the early beat is usually abnormal; QRS axis is normal in the absence of conducting system disease

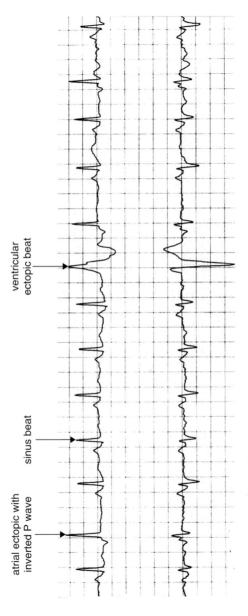

atrial ectopic with
inverted P wave

sinus beat

ventricular
ectopic beat

Sinus rhythm with atrial and ventricular ectopic beats

VENTRICULAR ECTOPICS

Regular/irregular rhythm	Regular with occasional early QRS. Ventricular bigeminy is when the ventricular ectopic beats (VEB) are paired with sinus beats in a repeating pattern
P waves present	Yes, on the normal sinus beats; there is no P wave prior to the ventricular ectopic
Atrial rate	Non-diagnostic
QRS rate	Non-diagnostic
P and QRS relationship	Non-diagnostic
PR interval	Normal, non-diagnostic
QRS width	Broad complex QRS on the ventricular ectopic beats
ST segments	Non-diagnostic
T waves	Non-diagnostic
Axis	Non-diagnostic

BIGEMINY

Atrial bigeminy, *see* atrial ectopics
Ventricular bigeminy, *see* ventricular ectopics

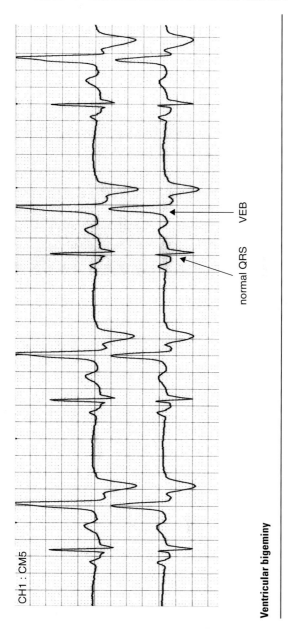

CH1 : CM5

VEB

normal QRS

Ventricular bigeminy

VENTRICULAR TACHYCARDIA

Regular/irregular rhythm	Regular
P waves present	Usually, no discernible P waves; occasionally, P waves can be seen in the T wave region if there is ventriculoatrial conduction. Often the atria still contract under control of the SA node while the ventricle is under the control of the ventricular tachycardia focus or circuit
Atrial rate	Not easily discernible
QRS rate	Over 100 per minute
P and QRS relationship	No standard pattern
PR interval	Non-diagnostic
QRS width	Wide complex; all wide complex regular tachycardias should on first inspection be regarded as ventricular tachycardia
ST segments	Non-diagnostic
T waves	Non-diagnostic
Axis	Non-diagnostic

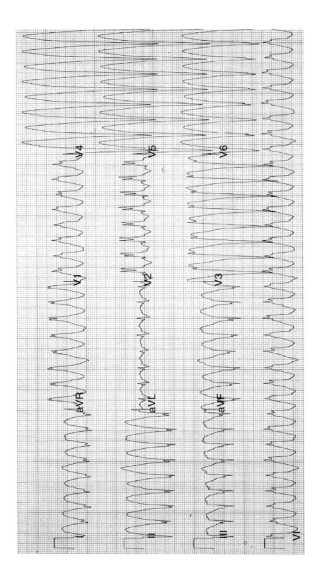

Ventricular tachycardia

3

SUPRAVENTRICULAR TACHYCARDIA

Regular/irregular rhythm	Regular
P waves present	Usually not visible, rarely may be seen between the QRS complexes
Atrial rate	If P waves visible the rate is equal to the ventricular rate
QRS rate	Usually between 160 and around 250 per minute
P and QRS relationship	Usually P waves are not visible but if they are present there is one P to each QRS
PR interval	Non-diagnostic
QRS width	Narrow complex, unless there is a ventricular conduction defect or antidromic SVT utilising an accessory pathway for conduction from atrium to ventricle. This uncommon type of SVT uses the atrioventricular node for the return path to the atrium
ST segments	Non-diagnostic, but ST depression is common with fast SVT
T waves	Non-diagnostic
Axis	Non-diagnostic

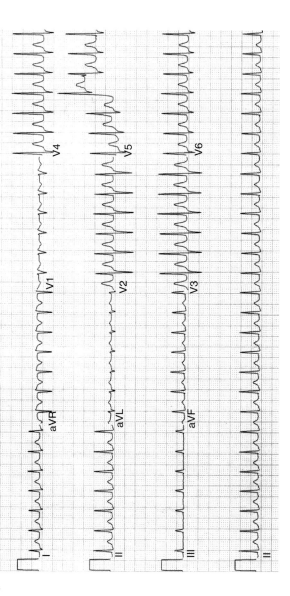

Supraventricular tachycardia

WOLFF-PARKINSON-WHITE SYNDROME

Regular/irregular rhythm	Non-diagnostic
P waves present	Yes
Atrial rate	Non-diagnostic
QRS rate	Non-diagnostic
P and QRS relationship	One P wave preceding each QRS
PR interval	Short
QRS width	QRS has a slurring of the upstroke of the R wave—this is the delta wave
ST segments	Non-diagnostic
T waves	Non-diagnostic
Axis	Non-diagnostic

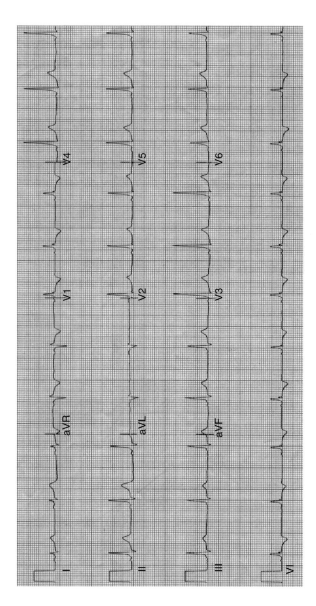

Sinus rhythm with Wolff-Parkinson-White syndrome

JUNCTIONAL RHYTHM

Regular/irregular rhythm	Regular
P waves present	Retrograde P waves may occur immediately before the QRS, within the QRS (invisible on surface ECG) or after the QRS
Atrial rate	If P waves are visible the rate is equal to the ventricular rate
QRS rate	40–80 per minute. Junctional rhythm is usually an escape rhythm when the sinus node fails and hence is usually slower than sinus rhythm
P and QRS relationship	If the P waves are visible there is one P for each QRS
PR interval	Non-diagnostic
QRS width	Normal or slightly prolonged
ST segments	Non-diagnostic
T waves	Non-diagnostic
Axis	Non-diagnostic

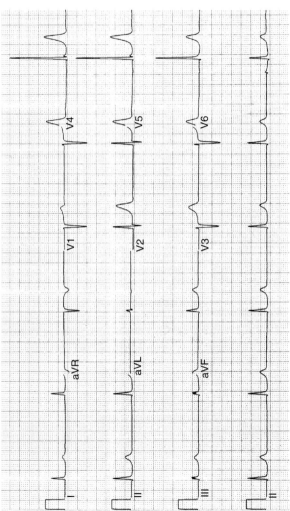

3

Junctional rhythm

LEFT BUNDLE BRANCH BLOCK (LBBB)

Regular/irregular rhythm	Non-diagnostic
P waves present	Non-diagnostic
Atrial rate	Non-diagnostic
QRS rate	Varies depending on the rhythm. If the rate is over 100 per minute and the rhythm is regular, be sure to check there are P waves present, as the main differential will be ventricular tachycardia. If the rhythm is over 100 per minute and irregularly irregular, it is most likely atrial fibrillation with bundle branch block
P and QRS relationship	Non-diagnostic
PR interval	Non-diagnostic
QRS width	Wide, > 3 small squares (0.12 s). There is either one or both of the following: QRS will have a W shape in V1 and/or an M shape in V6. The V1 complex is below the isoelectric line (negative), the V6 above it (positive). Remember, ask William Morrow (see page 72)
ST segments	Cannot be interpreted in the presence of bundle branch block
T waves	Cannot be interpreted in the presence of bundle branch block
Axis	Can be normal or, rarely, right axis deviation. Left axis deviation is otherwise common but is not caused by the LBBB

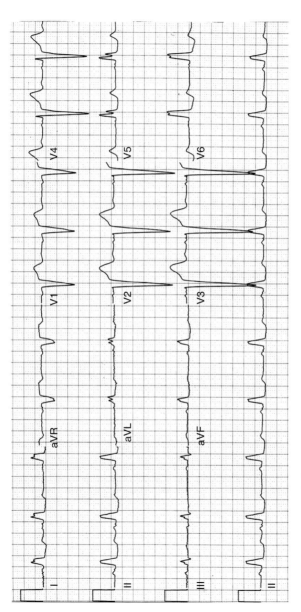

Sinus rhythm with left bundle branch block

RIGHT BUNDLE BRANCH BLOCK (RBBB)

Regular/irregular rhythm	Non-diagnostic
P waves present	Non-diagnostic
Atrial rate	Non-diagnostic
QRS rate	Varies depending on the rhythm. If the rate is over 100 per minute and the rhythm is regular, be sure to check there are P waves present, as the main differential will be ventricular tachycardia. If the rhythm is over 100 per minute and irregularly irregular, it is most likely atrial fibrillation with bundle branch block
P and QRS relationship	Non-diagnostic
PR interval	Non-diagnostic
QRS width	Wide, > 3 small squares (0.12 s). There is either one or both of the following: QRS will have an M shape in V1 and/or a W shape in V6. The V1 complex is above the isoelectric line (positive), the V6 below it (negative). Remember William Morrow (see page 72)
ST segments	Cannot be interpreted in the presence of bundle branch block
T waves	Cannot be interpreted in the presence of bundle branch block
Axis	Can be normal, or left or right deviation. If left axis deviation is present, check for left anterior hemiblock; this combination is common and is referred to as bifascicular block

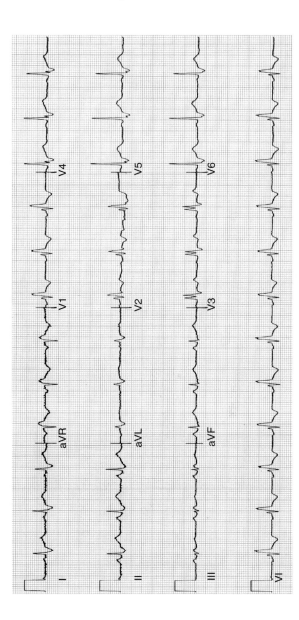

Sinus rhythm with right bundle branch block

RIGHT BUNDLE BRANCH BLOCK (PARTIAL)

Regular/irregular rhythm	Non-diagnostic
P waves present	Non-diagnostic
Atrial rate	Non-diagnostic
QRS rate	Non-diagnostic
P and QRS relationship	Non-diagnostic
PR interval	Non-diagnostic
QRS width	Between 0.10 and 0.12 seconds in duration. There is either one or both of the following: QRS will have an M shape in V1 and/or a W shape in V6. The V1 complex is above the isoelectric line (positive), the V6 below it (negative)
ST segments	Cannot be interpreted reliably in the presence of bundle branch block
T waves	Cannot be interpreted reliably in the presence of bundle branch block
Axis	Can be normal, or left or right deviation

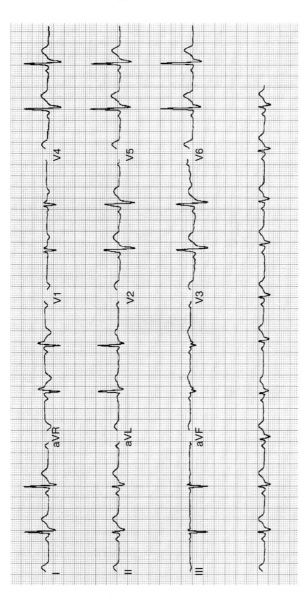

3

Sinus rhythm with partial right bundle branch block

LEFT ANTERIOR FASCICULAR (HEMI) BLOCK

Regular/irregular rhythm	Non-diagnostic
P waves present	Non-diagnostic
Atrial rate	Non-diagnostic
QRS rate	Non-diagnostic
P and QRS relationship	Non-diagnostic
PR interval	Non-diagnostic
QRS width	Normal width (if prolonged, check for coexisting RBBB). There is a characteristic pattern in the precordial leads: leads I and aVL are positive (often with a small initial Q); leads II, III, aVF are negative (with a small initial R wave). Left axis deviation, with QRS duration < 0.12 s, in the absence of transmural inferior infarction, is usually due to left anterior fascicular block
ST segments	Non-diagnostic
T waves	Non-diagnostic
Axis	Left axis deviation

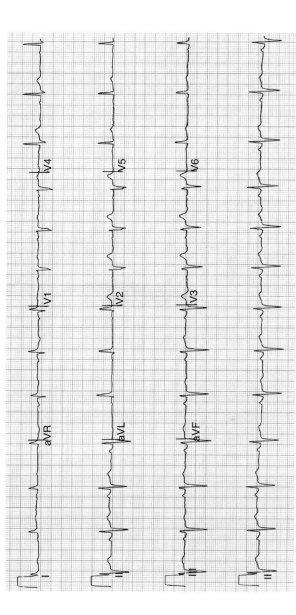

Sinus rhythm with left anterior fascicular block

LEFT POSTERIOR FASCICULAR (HEMI) BLOCK

Regular/irregular rhythm	Non-diagnostic
P waves present	Non-diagnostic
Atrial rate	Non-diagnostic
QRS rate	Non-diagnostic
P and QRS relationship	Non-diagnostic
PR interval	Non-diagnostic
QRS width	Normal width (if prolonged, check for coexisting RBBB). There is a characteristic pattern in the precordial leads: leads I and aVL are negative (often with a small initial R); leads II, III, aVF are positive (with a small initial Q wave). Right axis deviation, with QRS duration < 0.12 s, in the absence of transmural anterior infarction, is usually due to left posterior hemiblock
Axis	Right axis deviation

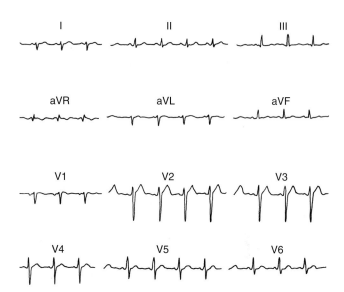

Sinus rhythm with left posterior fascicular block

ACUTE ANTERIOR MYOCARDIAL INFARCTION

Regular/irregular rhythm	Non-diagnostic
P waves present	Non-diagnostic
Atrial rate	Non-diagnostic
QRS rate	Non-diagnostic
P and QRS relationship	Non-diagnostic
PR interval	Non-diagnostic
QRS width	Non-diagnostic, unless a new bundle branch block develops. The combination of a bundle branch block with clinical and examination findings of infarction should be treated with the same relevance as classic ST elevation in this context
ST segments	Convex upwards elevation (in transmural ischaemia or infarction); 2 mm elevation in two successive leads V2 to V4 for anterior infarction—sometimes also referred to as anteroseptal infarction
T waves	Initially tall and peaked until the ST segments elevate to give the characteristic pattern
Axis	Non-diagnostic

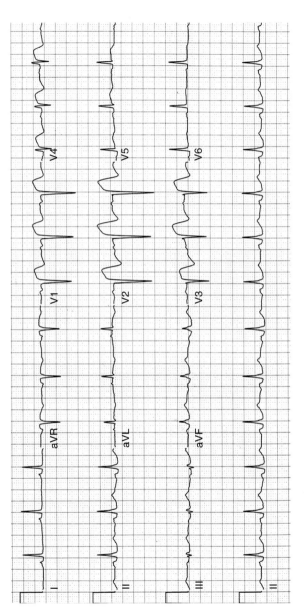

Sinus rhythm with acute anterior infarction

ACUTE ANTEROLATERAL MYOCARDIAL INFARCTION

Regular/irregular rhythm	Non-diagnostic
P waves present	Non-diagnostic
Atrial rate	Non-diagnostic
QRS rate	Non-diagnostic
P and QRS relationship	Non-diagnostic
PR interval	Non-diagnostic
QRS width	Non-diagnostic, unless a new bundle branch block develops. The combination of a bundle branch block with clinical and examination findings of infarction should be treated with the same relevance as classic ST elevation in this context
ST segments	Convex upwards elevation (in transmural ischaemia or infarction); 2 mm elevation in two successive leads V2 to V6 for anterolateral wall infarction. Pure lateral infarction is rare; it shows on the ECG as ST elevation localised to leads V5 and V6 (> 2 mm height), and occasionally the 'high lateral' leads, I and aVL (> 1 mm high)
T waves	Initially tall and peaked until the ST segments elevate to give the characteristic pattern
Axis	Non-diagnostic

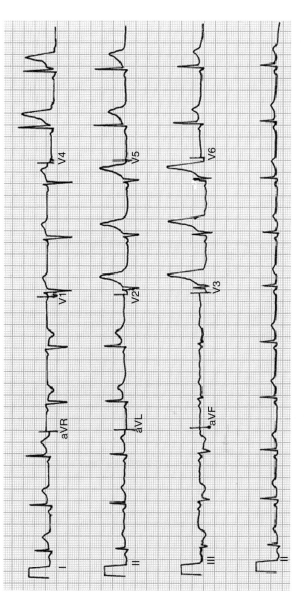

Sinus rhythm with acute anterolateral infarction

ACUTE INFERIOR MYOCARDIAL INFARCTION

Regular/irregular rhythm	Non-diagnostic
P waves present	Non-diagnostic
Atrial rate	Non-diagnostic
QRS rate	Non-diagnostic
P and QRS relationship	Non-diagnostic
PR interval	Non-diagnostic, but atrioventricular block is a frequent finding in acute inferior infarction
QRS width	Non-diagnostic, unless a new bundle branch block develops. The combination of a bundle branch block with clinical and examination findings of infarction should be treated with the same relevance as classic ST elevation in this context
ST segments	Convex upwards elevation (in transmural ischaemia or infarction); 1 mm of ST segment elevation in two of leads II, III or aVF for inferior wall infarction. Lateral extension of the ST elevation (leads V5, V6) is common. Look also for posterior extension of the infarct
T waves	Initially tall and peaked until the ST segments elevate to give the characteristic pattern
Axis	Non-diagnostic

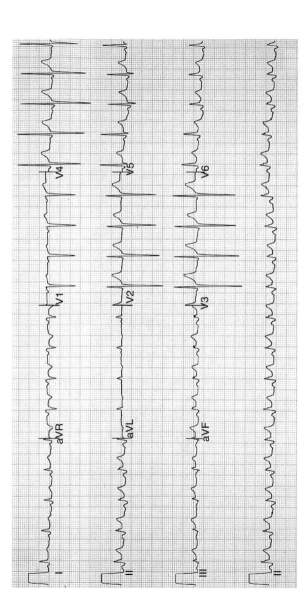

Sinus rhythm with acute inferior infarction

3

ACUTE POSTERIOR MYOCARDIAL INFARCTION

Regular/irregular rhythm	Non-diagnostic
P waves present	Non-diagnostic
Atrial rate	Non-diagnostic
QRS rate	Non-diagnostic
P and QRS relationship	Non-diagnostic
PR interval	Non-diagnostic
QRS width	Non-diagnostic, unless a new bundle branch block develops. The combination of a bundle branch block with clinical and examination findings of infarction should be treated with the same relevance as classic ST elevation in this context
ST segments	Convex downwards depression in leads V1 and V2. The V leads record electrical activity from the front of the heart. Electrical changes in the posterior wall are therefore seen as the opposite of the changes we see from anterior wall events. For this reason, ST depression indicates infarction of the posterior wall. Isolated posterior myocardial infarction is uncommon and posterior infarction is usually seen in combination with acute inferior infarction
T waves	May be T wave inversion
Axis	Non-diagnostic

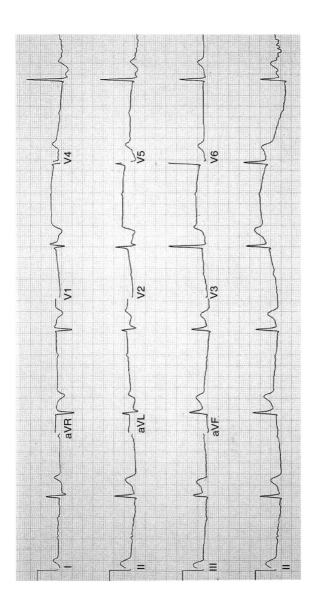

Complete atrioventricular block and acute inferoposterior infarction

OLD MYOCARDIAL INFARCTION

Regular/irregular rhythm	Non-diagnostic
P waves present	Non-diagnostic
Atrial rate	Non-diagnostic
QRS rate	Non-diagnostic
P and QRS relationship	Non-diagnostic
PR interval	Non-diagnostic
QRS width	Non-diagnostic; there will be pathological Q waves in leads overlying the infarcted territory. In the case of posterior infarction, an R wave will be present in V1 (the equivalent in meaning to a Q wave)
ST segments	In most patients they normalise by one week after infarction. If still elevated at one month, consider ventricular aneurysm formation
T waves	Normalise early in the infarction process; should be normal by one month in all patients post transmural infarction. Non-transmural or subendocardial infarction will have deep T wave inversion over the affected territory early in the recovery. In most cases, the T waves normalise by one month. There is no loss of R wave in non-transmural infarction
Axis	Non-diagnostic

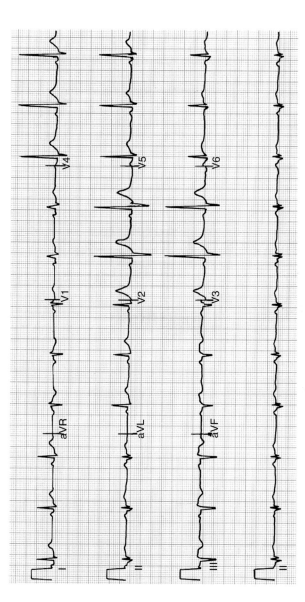

Sinus rhythm with previous (old) inferoposterior infarction

MYOCARDIAL ISCHAEMIA

Regular/irregular rhythm	Non-diagnostic
P waves present	Non-diagnostic
Atrial rate	Non-diagnostic
QRS rate	Non-diagnostic
P and QRS relationship	Non-diagnostic
PR interval	Non-diagnostic
QRS width	Non-diagnostic
ST segments	Depression of ST segments is the usual sign of non-transmural myocardial ischaemia or subendocardial infarction. As a rule of thumb, the deeper the ST depression the more significant the ischaemia. If present during chest pain, the specificity of ST depression is further improved
T waves	T wave inversion can occur during ischaemia
Axis	Non-diagnostic

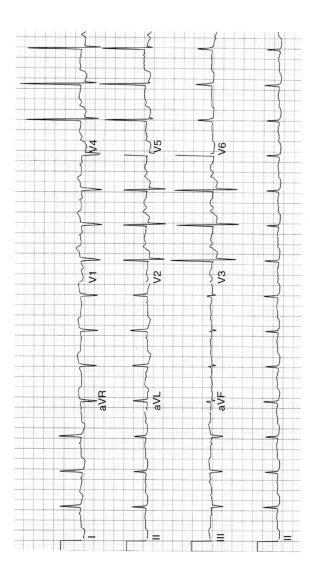

Sinus rhythm with anterolateral ischaemic ST depression

FIRST-DEGREE ATRIOVENTRICULAR BLOCK

Regular/irregular rhythm	Non-diagnostic
P waves present	Yes
Atrial rate	Non-diagnostic
QRS rate	Non-diagnostic
P and QRS relationship	A P wave preceding each QRS complex
PR interval	Prolonged, > 5 small squares (> 0.20 seconds)
QRS width	Non-diagnostic
ST segments	Non-diagnostic
T waves	Non-diagnostic
Axis	Non-diagnostic

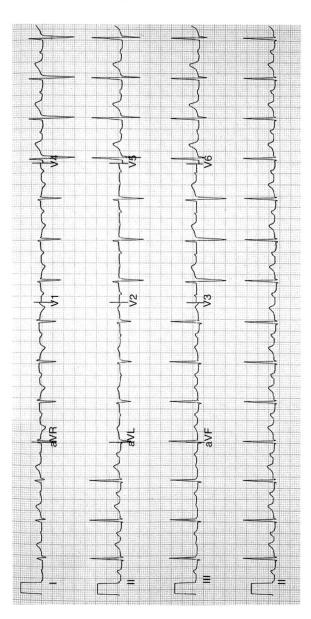

Sinus rhythm with first-degree atrioventricular block

SECOND-DEGREE ATRIOVENTRICULAR BLOCK (MOBITZ TYPE 1, WENCKEBACH PHENOMENON)

Regular/irregular rhythm	Non-diagnostic, but usually regularly irregular
P waves present	Yes
Atrial rate	Greater than ventricular rate
QRS rate	Non-diagnostic
P and QRS relationship	A P wave preceding most QRS complexes
PR interval	Becomes longer with each beat until a P wave fails to conduct and a QRS is dropped. After the dropped beat, conduction resumes and the pattern recommences
QRS width	Non-diagnostic
ST segments	Non-diagnostic
T waves	Non-diagnostic
Axis	Non-diagnostic

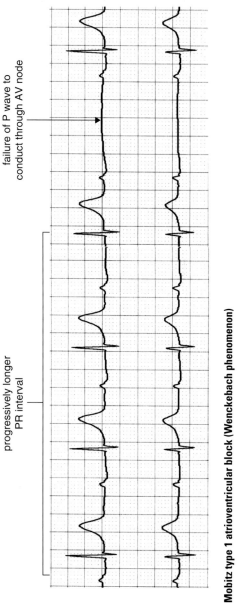

failure of P wave to
conduct through AV node

progressively longer
PR interval

Mobitz type 1 atrioventricular block (Wenckebach phenomenon)

SECOND-DEGREE ATRIOVENTRICULAR BLOCK (MOBITZ TYPE 2)

Regular/irregular rhythm	Non-diagnostic
P waves present	Yes
Atrial rate	Greater than ventricular rate
QRS rate	Non-diagnostic
P and QRS relationship	There is a ratio (occasionally variable) of P waves to QRS complexes, usually 2:1
PR interval	Can be either normal or prolonged on the beats that conduct to the ventricle
QRS width	Non-diagnostic
ST segments	Non-diagnostic
T waves	Non-diagnostic
Axis	Non-diagnostic

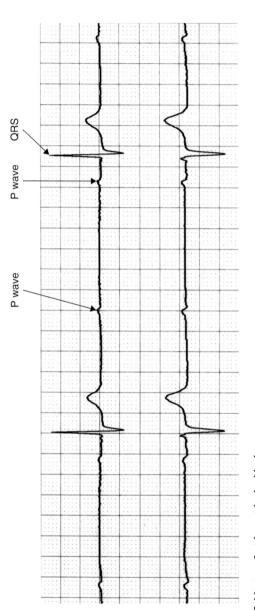

QRS

P wave

P wave

Mobitz type 2 atrioventricular block

THIRD-DEGREE ATRIOVENTRICULAR BLOCK (COMPLETE HEART BLOCK)

Regular/irregular rhythm	Non-diagnostic
P waves present	Yes
Atrial rate	Greater than ventricular rate
QRS rate	Non-diagnostic, but usually a bradycardia (< 60 bpm)
P and QRS relationship	No regular relationship
PR interval	Non-diagnostic
QRS width	Non-diagnostic, but in most cases wider than normal as the escape rhythm comes from the atrioventricular junction or ventricular muscle. Generally, the lower in the heart the escape rhythm originates, the slower the response and the wider the QRS
ST segments	Non-diagnostic
T waves	Non-diagnostic
Axis	Non-diagnostic

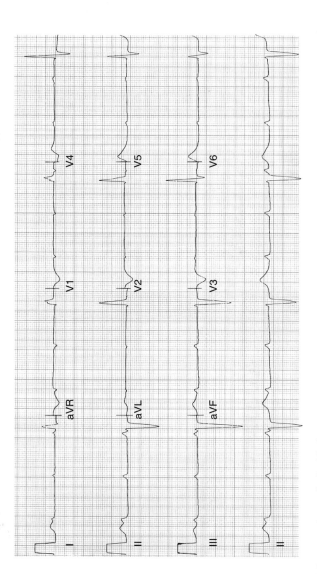

Third-degree atrioventricular block

RIGHT VENTRICULAR HYPERTROPHY

Regular/irregular rhythm	Non-diagnostic
P waves present	Yes, may be right atrial hypertrophy (P pulmonale)
Atrial rate	Non-diagnostic
QRS rate	Non-diagnostic
P and QRS relationship	Non-diagnostic
PR interval	Non-diagnostic
QRS width	Non-diagnostic, but there is a characteristic pattern: the R waves are tall in II, III and V1 (> 7 mm or ≥ S wave depth in V1); the S waves are relatively deeper in V4 to V6 and, if there is right ventricular dilatation, the S waves are the dominant part of the QRS across all the V leads
ST segments	Often ST depression in II, III, aVF and V1
T waves	Often T wave inversion in II, III, aVF and V1
Axis	Right axis deviation

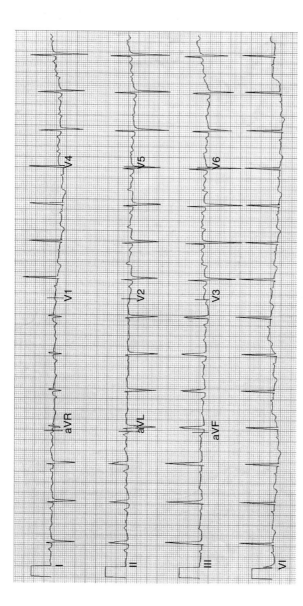

Right ventricular hypertrophy

LEFT VENTRICULAR HYPERTROPHY

Regular/irregular rhythm	Non-diagnostic
P waves present	Non-diagnostic, but left atrial enlargement (P mitrale) may be present
Atrial rate	Non-diagnostic
QRS rate	Non-diagnostic
P and QRS relationship	Non-diagnostic
PR interval	Non-diagnostic
QRS width	Non-diagnostic, but the diagnosis is made based on the QRS voltages. The R wave in V1 + S wave in V5 > 35 mm, or R wave in V2 + S wave in V6 > 35 mm, or an R wave > 20 mm in lead I, or S wave > 20 mm in III
ST segments	Non-diagnostic, but the finding of ST segment depression in the lateral leads, V5 and V6, is common and occasionally reported as a 'strain pattern'. The ST depression is often downsloping and the R wave, ST-T, is said to look like a hockey stick
T waves	Non-diagnostic
Axis	Non-diagnostic, but left axis deviation may be present

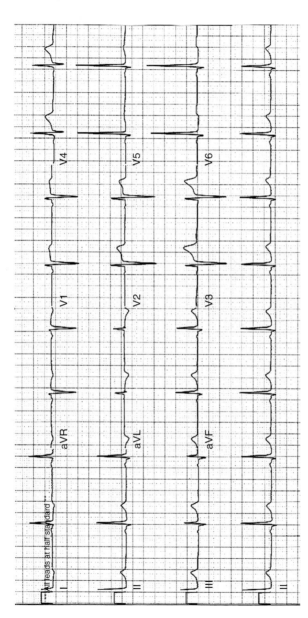

All leads at half standard

I

aVR

V1

V4

II

aVL

V2

V5

III

aVF

V3

V6

II

Sinus rhythm with half calibration and left ventricular hypertrophy

PERICARDITIS

Regular/irregular rhythm	Non-diagnostic
P waves present	Yes
Atrial rate	Non-diagnostic
QRS rate	Non-diagnostic
P and QRS relationship	Non-diagnostic
PR interval	Non-diagnostic, but depression of the PR segment below the isoelectric line is often seen
QRS width	Non-diagnostic. In the presence of a bundle branch block the ST segments cannot be interpreted and hence pericarditis cannot be diagnosed via ECG criteria
ST segments	Pericarditis is difficult to diagnose confidently on ECG criteria alone. Usually, the ST elevation is horizontal or concave upward, and widespread throughout all leads, although in some cases it can be localised. There is usually still a distinction between the ST segment and T wave
T waves	Non-diagnostic
Axis	Non-diagnostic

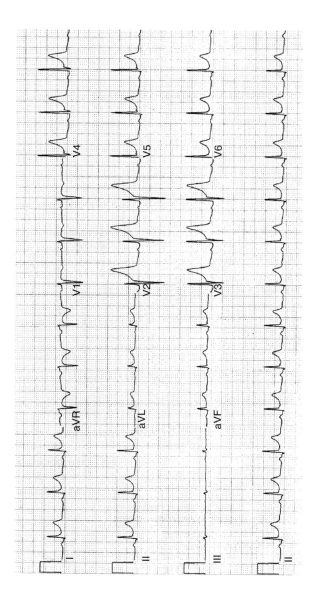

Sinus rhythm with widespread ST elevation consistent with pericarditis

PERICARDIAL EFFUSION

Regular/irregular rhythm	Non-diagnostic
P waves present	Non-diagnostic
Atrial rate	Non-diagnostic
QRS rate	Non-diagnostic
P and QRS relationship	Non-diagnostic
PR interval	Non-diagnostic
QRS width	The width is non-diagnostic but the height of the complexes makes the diagnosis. The voltages recorded in the V leads are much smaller that usual; this low voltage pattern is highly suggestive of pericardial fluid. QRS alternans is also occasionally seen—this is when the QRS complex varies in height with each beat, usually a pattern of smaller voltage, higher voltage, smaller voltage etc. with each beat. This is due to the pendulum-like motion of the heart within the fluid-filled pericardial space, coming closer to the anterior chest wall with one beat and then closer to the posterior wall with the next beat, giving a lower voltage signal
ST segments	Non-diagnostic
T waves	Non-diagnostic
Axis	Non-diagnostic

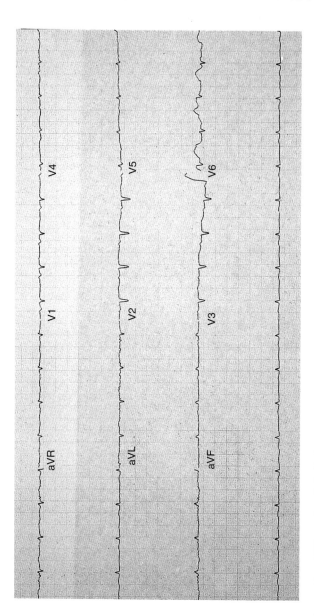

Low voltage ECG—pericardial effusion

SECTION 4

PACEMAKERS
AND ECGs

Pacemakers are becoming more prevalent as they become smaller and easier to insert. The indications for insertion of a pacemaker are continually broadening as new technologies emerge.

The interpretation of an ECG in a patient with a pacemaker requires some understanding of these devices and the ECG changes they can produce. The ECG may also give information as to whether a pacemaker is working correctly.

PACEMAKERS

These devices were originally designed to prevent bradycardias. They consist of a pulse generator that is surgically implanted, usually in the anterior chest under the clavicle, and a lead or leads that go via the veins under the clavicle down into the heart. They monitor the spontaneous electrical activity of the heart and if a beat does not occur within a preset time interval an electrical pulse is sent down the wire to stimulate the heart and deliver the missing heartbeat.

Pacemakers have the capacity to synchronise atrial and ventricular contraction, they can increase the heart rate when they sense the patient is exercising and they have the capacity to store what has happened recently in their memory.

There are also pacemakers that are used for fast heart rhythms, namely ventricular tachycardia and ventricular fibrillation. These devices are larger and have the capacity to deliver a DC shock into the heart to revert it back to sinus rhythm if one of these malignant rhythms occurs.

Problems with anti-bradycardia pacemakers and the ECG

Filters
ECG machines and cardiac monitors have filters in them to remove electrical interference. These filters can sometimes remove, or filter out, the pacing spike from the ECG. If a patient has a pacemaker and you cannot see any spikes from pacing, turn off the muscle filter and then the 50 Hz filter to see if any spikes are evident. If you do not see any it is most likely that the patient is in spontaneous rhythm and the pacemaker is just monitoring and not pacing.

Intensive and coronary care monitoring units also often have a setting to enhance the pacing spikes. These can lead to problems with 'oversensing', that is putting spikes on the monitor when there is no pacing. Always confirm spikes on a monitor by doing a 12 lead ECG to check if they are really there.

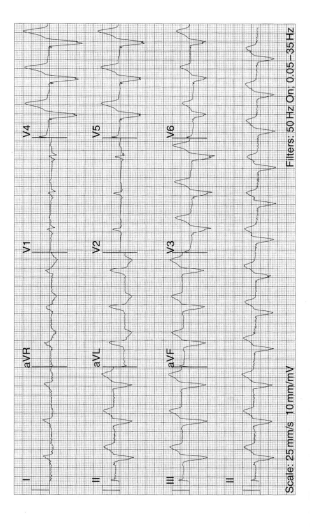

Scale: 25 mm/s 10 mm/mV

Filters: 50 Hz On: 0.05–35 Hz

ECG with the filters activated—difficult to see any pacing spikes

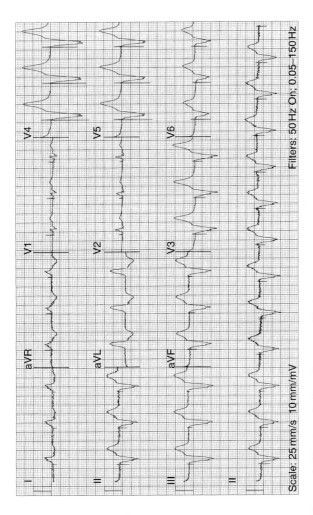

Scale: 25 mm/s 10 mm/mV

Filters: 50Hz On; 0.05–150Hz

ECG with the muscle filter turned off—spikes are evident

ECG pattern

The leads from the pacemaker are sited into the right atrial append-age in the case of atrial leads and into the right ventricular apex for ventricular leads. Pacing via the atrial lead gives a P wave that is similar in morphology to a spontaneous P wave. Pacing via the lead in the right ventricular apex however, activates the ventricles from the bottom up and hence gives an abnormal QRS. The QRS pattern should be of left bundle branch morphology. A right bundle branch pattern after implantation can mean that the ventricular pacing wire is in the coronary sinus or in the left ventricle via a patent foramen ovale, septal perforation or perforation into the pericardial space.

Electrical capture of myocardium

For the pacemaker to work it needs to deliver an electrical impulse to the myocardium to initiate depolarisation. When depolarisation does not occur, it can be due to failure of the pulse generator, a problem in the lead such as a fracture, displacement of the lead so that the tip is floating free in the cavity or fibrosis around the tip of the lead imped-ing conduction to the muscle. Failure of capture of the myocardium is manifest on the ECG as a pacing spike but no subsequent electrical activity from the heart.

Sensing when to put in a paced beat

A critical function of pacemakers is knowing when to put in a paced beat. The pacemaker does this by monitoring the electrical activity of the heart via the leads. There are two main ways a pacemaker can make an error with sensing the spontaneous electrical activity. Oversensing is where it picks up other electrical activity and interprets it as a spon-taneous beat, thereby not putting in a paced beat when one is needed. Undersensing is where the pacemaker fails to detect a spontaneous beat and puts in a pulse when it is not required. Oversensing can lead to syncope if the patient is pacemaker reliant whereas undersensing can lead to pacing on a T wave and inducing ventricular fibrillation.

Fusion of pacing and spontaneous beats

Fusion occurs when the intrinsic heart rate is the same as the mini-mum heart rate set on the pacemaker. The pacemaker senses a beat, waits the preset interval for the next beat, then delivers a pulse. During the time from when the pacemaker senses a beat is necessary to delivering one there is spontaneous activation of the heart, giving an ECG complex that is a combination of both stimuli, or a spontane-ous complex with a pacing spike in the QRS (due to the pacing spike not capturing as the muscle is already depolarising).

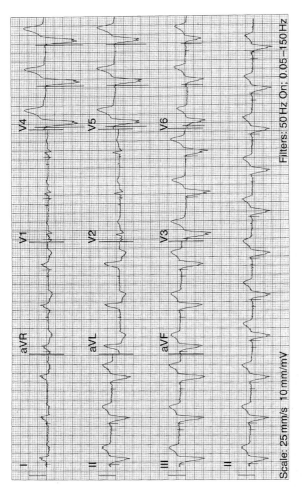

Scale: 25 mm/s 10 mm/mV   Filters: 50 Hz On; 0.05–150 Hz

Failure of capture of the atrial pacing impulse

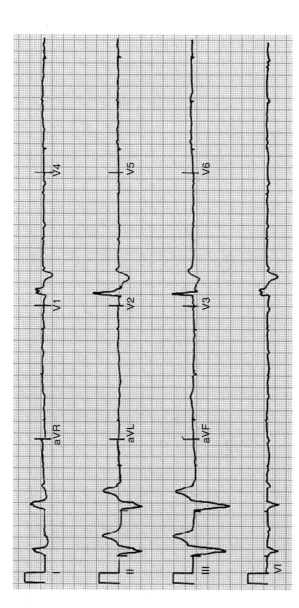

Failure of capture of the ventricular pacing impulse

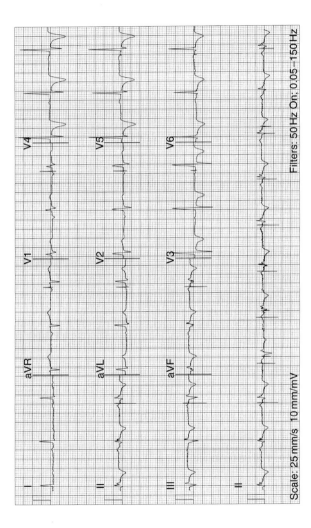

Scale: 25 mm/s 10 mm/mV

Filters: 50 Hz On: 0.05–150 Hz

Failure of sensing for both the atrial and ventricular leads. The pacing spikes are at times occurring on the P wave and within or after the QRS complexes

Dual chamber pacing and the ECG

When a patient has a dual chamber pacemaker, the atrial and ventricular leads function independently in that they each sense and pace their own chambers according to need. The delay between the atrial and ventricular pacing can also be set, providing customised AV delay.

Depending on the site of the patient's conduction disease, one or other mode of pacing may predominate. If they have sinus nodal disease and normal atrioventricular conduction then the atrial lead will do most of the pacing whereas if they have a normal sinus node and atrioventricular disease, the P waves will be spontaneous and the subsequent ventricular activation will be from the pacemaker.

There are times where no pacing is needed and other times where one or both chambers are actively pacing.

4

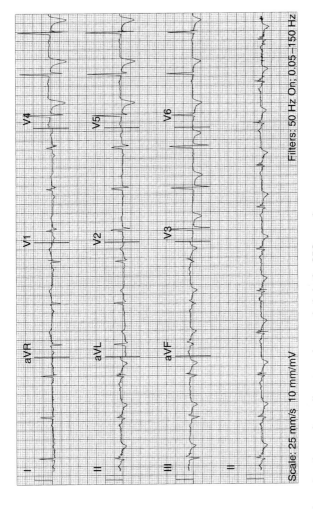

Scale: 25 mm/s 10 mm/mV

Filters: 50 Hz On; 0.05–150 Hz

Failure of sensing, the pacing spike appearing regularly in the QRS complex

INDEX